The Effect of Diet and Natural Agents on Oral, Periodontal Health and Dentistry

The Effect of Diet and Natural Agents on Oral, Periodontal Health and Dentistry

Editor

Gaetano Isola

MDPI • Basel • Beijing • Wuhan • Barcelona • Belgrade • Manchester • Tokyo • Cluj • Tianjin

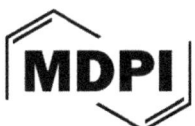

Editor
Gaetano Isola
Department of General Surgery
and Surgical-Medical Specialties,
School of Dentistry,
University of Catania
Italy

Editorial Office
MDPI
St. Alban-Anlage 66
4052 Basel, Switzerland

This is a reprint of articles from the Special Issue published online in the open access journal *Nutrients* (ISSN 2072-6643) (available at: https://www.mdpi.com/journal/nutrients/special_issues/Diet_Dentistry).

For citation purposes, cite each article independently as indicated on the article page online and as indicated below:

LastName, A.A.; LastName, B.B.; LastName, C.C. Article Title. *Journal Name* **Year**, *Article Number*, Page Range.

ISBN 978-3-03943-511-1 (Hbk)
ISBN 978-3-03943-512-8 (PDF)

© 2020 by the authors. Articles in this book are Open Access and distributed under the Creative Commons Attribution (CC BY) license, which allows users to download, copy and build upon published articles, as long as the author and publisher are properly credited, which ensures maximum dissemination and a wider impact of our publications.

The book as a whole is distributed by MDPI under the terms and conditions of the Creative Commons license CC BY-NC-ND.

Contents

About the Editor vii

Gaetano Isola
The Impact of Diet, Nutrition and Nutraceuticals on Oral and Periodontal Health
Reprinted from: *Nutrients* 2020, *12*, 2724, doi:10.3390/nu12092724 1

Gaetano Isola
Current Evidence of Natural Agents in Oral and Periodontal Health
Reprinted from: *Nutrients* 2020, *12*, 585, doi:10.3390/nu12020585 7

Zhibin Liu, Hongwen Guo, Wen Zhang and Li Ni
Salivary Microbiota Shifts under Sustained Consumption of Oolong Tea in Healthy Adults
Reprinted from: *Nutrients* 2020, *12*, 966, doi:10.3390/nu12040966 11

Gaetano Isola, Alessandro Polizzi, Simone Muraglie, Rosalia Leonardi and Antonino Lo Giudice
Assessment of vitamin C and Antioxidant Profiles in Saliva and Serum in Patients with Periodontitis and Ischemic Heart Disease
Reprinted from: *Nutrients* 2019, *11*, 2956, doi:10.3390/nu11122956 27

Aiste Jekabsone, Inga Sile, Andrea Cochis, Marina Makrecka-Kuka, Goda Laucaityte, Elina Makarova, Lia Rimondini, Rasa Bernotiene, Lina Raudone, Evelina Vedlugaite, Rasa Baniene, Alina Smalinskiene, Nijole Savickiene and Maija Dambrova
Investigation of Antibacterial and Antiinflammatory Activities of Proanthocyanidins from *Pelargonium sidoides* DC Root Extract
Reprinted from: *Nutrients* 2019, *11*, 2829, doi:10.3390/nu11112829 41

Maria Bogdan, Andreea Daniela Meca, Mihail Virgil Boldeanu, Dorin Nicolae Gheorghe, Adina Turcu-Stiolica, Mihaela-Simona Subtirelu, Lidia Boldeanu, Mihaela Blaj, Gina Eosefina Botnariu, Cristiana Elena Vlad, Liliana Georgeta Foia and Petra Surlin
Possible Involvement of Vitamin C in Periodontal Disease-Diabetes Mellitus Association
Reprinted from: *Nutrients* 2020, *12*, 553, doi:10.3390/nu12020553 59

Livia Nastri, Antimo Moretti, Silvia Migliaccio, Marco Paoletta, Marco Annunziata, Sara Liguori, Giuseppe Toro, Massimiliano Bianco, Gennaro Cecoro, Luigi Guida and Giovanni Iolascon
Do Dietary Supplements and Nutraceuticals Have Effects on Dental Implant Osseointegration? A Scoping Review
Reprinted from: *Nutrients* 2020, *12*, 268, doi:10.3390/nu12010268 77

About the Editor

Gaetano Isola is an Assistant Professor at the University of Catania, Catania, Italy. He qualified in Dentistry in 2009 at the University of Messina, Italy. He completed his Ph.D. in "Physiopathology of the Stomatognathic Apparatus and Dental Materials" at the University of Turin, Turin, Italy. He was a visiting Research Fellow at the "Laboratory the Study of Calcified Tissues and Biomaterials" at the Department of Periodontology Université de Montréal, Canada, Advanced Course in Periodontology at the University of Ferrara, the Master Course in Periodontology at the University of Verona, and the three-year certificate in Oral Surgery at the University of Naples "Federico II". He was a Visiting Professor at the Department of Periodontology at the University of North Carolina at Chapel Hill, USA and the Department of Oral Surgery of the University of Granada, Spain. He was a Visiting Researcher at the Department of Implantology and Oral Surgery at the University of Bern, Switzerland, and the Department of Periodontology of the "Eastman Dental Institute", London. He also obtained the National Scientific Qualification of Associate Professor for the Academic Discipline of Odontostomatology, Sector 06/F1, Italian Minister of University and Research (MIUR). Dr. Isola has been a recipient of many research awards, among others the "Global Peer Review Awards" of the Web of Science Group, and the "Travel Grant Award 2020" and "Outstanding Reviewer Award 2019" from MDPI Publishing, and he was selected for the "IADR Robert Frank Junior Award" CED-IADR/NOF Oral Health Research Association and the "USERN 2020 award", Universal Scientific Education and Research Network (USERN). He is an active member of the Italian Society of Oral Surgery (SIdCO) and the International Piezoelectric Surgery Academy (IPA). He is a Board Member of the International Association of Dental Research (IADR) and a member of the Italian Society of Periodontology (SIdP). He is also an active member of the "International IADR Constitution Committee" of the International Association of Dental Research (IADR) (2016–2019 and 2019–2022). He has served as an advisor for several research projects and has been a speaker at national and international Periodontology and Oral Surgery conferences. He is an author of over 100 national and international peer-reviewed publications. His main research interests focus on the clinical, biological, and pharmacological aspects of periodontitis, and the relationship between oral health and systemic health.

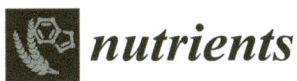

Editorial

The Impact of Diet, Nutrition and Nutraceuticals on Oral and Periodontal Health

Gaetano Isola

Department of General Surgery and Surgical-Medical Specialties, School of Dentistry, University of Catania, Via S. Sofia 78, 95124 Catania, Italy; gaetano.isola@unict.it; Tel.: +39-095-3782453

Received: 21 August 2020; Accepted: 28 August 2020; Published: 6 September 2020

Abstract: Oral and periodontal diseases can determine severe functional, phonatory and aesthetic impairments and are the main cause of adult tooth loss. They are caused by some specific bacteria that provoke an intense local inflammatory response and affect—with particular gravity—susceptible subjects, because of reasons related to genetics and lifestyles (e.g., smoking and home oral hygiene habits). They are more frequent in the disadvantaged segments of society and, in particular, in subjects who have difficulty accessing preventive services and dental care. Some systemic diseases, such as uncontrolled diabetes, can increase their risk of development and progression. Recently, in addition to the obvious considerations of severe alterations and impairments for oral health and well-being, it has been noted that periodontitis can cause changes in the whole organism. Numerous clinical and experimental studies have highlighted the presence of a strong association between periodontitis and some systemic diseases, in particular, cardiovascular diseases, diabetes, lung diseases and complications of pregnancy. The purpose of this editorial is to provide a current and thoughtful perspective on the relationship of diet and natural agents on oral, periodontal diseases, and chewing disorder preventions which may reflect good systemic conditions and related quality of life or to analyze indirect effects through the contribution of diet and nutrition to systemic health in order to obtain a modern diagnostic–therapeutic approach.

Keywords: periodontitis; oral diseases; diet; nutrients; nutraceutics; therapy; host response

---

Editorial

Periodontitis is a multifactorial disease in which both environmental and genetic factors play a precise and controversial role in determining its onset [1]. Oral bacterial flora certainly plays an important role in the progression of this pathology. Further risk factors, widely studied, are smoking and diabetes [2–4]. However, a series of genetic factors of the host can condition the individual susceptibility to the onset of the disease, determine its different clinical manifestations and the rate of progression [5,6].

Unlike Mendelian genetic diseases, which are rare and caused by a single or few mutations, multifactorial diseases, such as periodontitis, are frequent and related to numerous environmental and genetic factors. Genetic factors are not real mutations, but genetic polymorphisms, also called susceptibility factors. Each of these is not necessary or sufficient to determine the disease, however, they are able to modify the risk of its onset [7,8].

These polymorphisms are variations in the genetic code that can have different effects, for example, changing the levels of gene expression, causing slight functional changes of the coded molecules, making individuals more susceptible to the onset of a certain disease or to the appearance of clinical pictures more serious than the disease itself [9].

In recent years, investigations into susceptibility factors for the development of periodontal diseases have mainly focused on the study of genes that encode factors involved in modulating the immune response, cell surface receptors, chemokines, enzymes and proteins related to antigen recognition. Cytokines, such as IL-1A, IL-1B, IL-10 and IL-6, are key factors that mediate the inflammatory process in periodontal disease. They play a role in the activation, proliferation and differentiation of B cells, the main cells implicated in severe manifestations of periodontitis [10–13].

These genetic variations can, therefore, favour the progression of the disease, causing the classic trend, characterized by repeated cycles of tissue inflammation, followed by spontaneous remissions (defined as "pousses" trend) [14,15].

In periodontal disease, pathogenic bacteria accumulated in the subgingival sulcus are the environmental factors that influence the inflammatory response of the periodontal tissues [16,17]. However, a central role of diet, natural agents and nutraceutics are also considered indirectly responsible for the health of periodontal tissues and against alveolar bone resorption [18–22].

In this regard, Liu et al. [23] found that seven bacterial taxa, including Streptococcus sp., Ruminococcaceae sp., Haemophilus sp., Veillonella spp., Actinomyces odontolyticus, and Gemella haemolysans, were significantly altered after oolong tea consumption, and presented robust strong connections with other oral microbiota. These results suggest that sustained oolong tea consumption would modulate salivary microbiota and generate potential oral pathogen preventative benefits.

Since alveolar bone resorption is a key factor in periodontal disease, the vitamin D receptor (VDR) has been considered as a susceptibility factor in disease progression. Data in the literature support the existence of an association between common polymorphisms affecting candidate genes and periodontal disease [22,24,25].

Interestingly, most genetic studies of periodontitis have employed small cohorts. The limited statistical power of studies conducted with a low number of samples leads to an imprecise assessment of the level of genetic risk and the danger of obtaining false-positive and false-negative results.

Periodontitis develops severely in genetically predisposed individuals [26,27]. Genetic susceptibility is believed to be due to changes in the subject's genes that lead to (i) a lower efficiency of the immune system in controlling the growth of pathogenic bacteria; and/or (ii) an imperfect regulation of the inflammatory response [28–32] which leads to an increase in the destructive side effects of inflammation [33–36]. As a matter of fact, Jekabsone et al. [37] explored antibacterial, antinflammatory and cytoprotective capacity of Pelargonium sidoides DC root extract (PSRE) and proanthocyanidin fraction from PSRE (PACN) under conditions characteristic for periodontal disease. They found that PSRE and especially PACN possess strong antibacterial, anti-inflammatory and gingival tissue protecting properties under periodontitis-mimicking conditions and are suggestable candidates for the treatment of periodontal disease.

Great importance is also attached to lifestyles [38]; first of all, smoking and home oral hygiene habits, orthodontic treatment [39–42] and malocclusions [43–48], as they explain at an epidemiological level a large portion of the cases of periodontitis and dental malocclusions [49–51] observed and are modifiable and therefore important for prevention and treatment.

The general state of health of the subject is another element that can increase the risk of developing periodontitis. For example, people with poorly controlled diabetes have three times higher risk than non-diabetics of developing periodontitis [52,53].

Bodgdan et al. [54] conducted a systematic review of clinical trials that measured plasmatic/salivary levels of ascorbic acid in PD–diabetes mellitus (DM) association. They found that decreased levels of vitamin C were observed in PD patients with DM but data about the efficacy of vitamin C administration are inconclusive. Given the important bidirectional relationship between PD and DM, there is a strong need for more research to assess the positive effects of ascorbic acid supplementation in individuals suffering from both diseases and also its proper regimen for these patients.

Moreover, in this aspect, Nastri et al. [55], in their scoping review, summarized the role of dietary supplements in optimizing osseointegration after implant insertion surgery. The authors concluded highlighting the limited role of nutraceuticals in promoting the osseointegration of dental implants.

However, in some cases, such as for vitamin D deficiency, there is a clear link among their deficit, reduced osseointegration, and early implant failure, thus requiring an adequate supplementation.

Knowing the patient's genetic profile or their predisposition to the disease could be very useful in diagnosing periodontal disease and in defining a personalized therapeutic plan. In addition, it could give prognostic indications of the outcome of the disease.

Data derived from epidemiological observations are therefore important to establish the existence of a relevant and stable association but are insufficient to demonstrate the causal link and therefore the general health benefits deriving from the treatment and prevention of periodontitis. Causality can only be demonstrated unequivocally in randomized controlled trials that include eliminating or reducing (through prevention or therapy) the exposure of subjects to the harmful effects of periodontitis: pathogenic bacteria and gingival inflammation. These studies must conform to the highest quality standards and test the therapy capable of reducing the exposure in a clinically relevant way for each systemic pathology for which a significant association has emerged.

Funding: This research received no external funding.

Conflicts of Interest: The author declares no conflict of interest.

References

1. Aarabi, G.; Heydecke, G.; Seedorf, U. Roles of Oral Infections in the Pathomechanism of Atherosclerosis. *Int. J. Mol. Sci.* **2018**, *19*. [CrossRef]
2. Decker, A.; Askar, H.; Tattan, M.; Taichman, R.; Wang, H.L. The assessment of stress, depression, and inflammation as a collective risk factor for periodontal diseases: A systematic review. *Clin. Oral Investig.* **2020**, *24*, 1–12. [CrossRef] [PubMed]
3. Almeida, M.L.; Duarte, P.M.; Figueira, E.A.; Lemos, J.C.; Nobre, C.M.G.; Miranda, T.S.; de Vasconcelos Gurgel, B.C. Effects of a full-mouth disinfection protocol on the treatment of type-2 diabetic and non diabetic subjects with mild-to-moderate periodontitis: One-year clinical outcomes. *Clin. Oral Investig.* **2020**, *24*, 333–341. [CrossRef] [PubMed]
4. Han, S.J.; Yi, Y.J.; Bae, K.H. The association between periodontitis and dyslipidemia according to smoking and harmful alcohol use in a representative sample of Korean adults. *Clin. Oral Investig.* **2020**, *24*, 937–944. [CrossRef]
5. Tonetti, M.S.; Greenwell, H.; Kornman, K.S. Staging and grading of periodontitis: Framework and proposal of a new classification and case definition. *J. Periodontol.* **2018**, *89* (Suppl. S1), S159–S172. [CrossRef] [PubMed]
6. Marra, P.M.; Nucci, L.; Femiano, L.; Grassia, V.; Nastri, L.; Perillo, L. Orthodontic management of a mandibular double-tooth incisor: A case report. *Open Dent. J.* **2020**, *14*, 219–255. [CrossRef]
7. Tasdemir, I.; Erbak Yilmaz, H.; Narin, F.; Saglam, M. Assessment of saliva and gingival crevicular fluid soluble urokinase plasminogen activator receptor (suPAR), galectin-1, and TNF-alpha levels in periodontal health and disease. *J. Periodontal. Res.* **2020**, *55*, 622–630. [CrossRef]
8. Duarte, P.M.; de Lorenzo Abreu, L.; Vilela, A.; Feres, M.; Giro, G.; Miranda, T.S. Protein and mRNA detection of classic cytokines in corresponding samples of serum, gingival tissue and gingival crevicular fluid from subjects with periodontitis. *J. Periodontal. Res.* **2019**, *54*, 174–179. [CrossRef]
9. Nisha, K.J.; Janam, P.; Harshakumar, K. Identification of a novel salivary biomarker miR-143-3p for periodontal diagnosis: A proof of concept study. *J. Periodontol.* **2019**, *90*, 1149–1159. [CrossRef]
10. Isola, G.; Polizzi, A.; Santonocito, S.; Alibrandi, A.; Ferlito, S. Expression of Salivary and Serum Malondialdehyde and Lipid Profile of Patients with Periodontitis and Coronary Heart Disease. *Int. J. Mol. Sci.* **2019**, *20*. [CrossRef]
11. Isola, G.; Alibrandi, A.; Rapisarda, E.; Matarese, G.; Williams, R.C.; Leonardi, R. Association of vitamin D in patients with periodontitis: A cross-sectional study. *J. Periodontal. Res.* **2020**, *55*, 602–612. [CrossRef] [PubMed]
12. Ghotloo, S.; Motedayyen, H.; Amani, D.; Saffari, M.; Sattari, M. Assessment of microRNA-146a in generalized aggressive periodontitis and its association with disease severity. *J. Periodontal. Res.* **2019**, *54*, 27–32. [CrossRef] [PubMed]

13. Marchetti, E.; Tecco, S.; Caterini, E.; Casalena, F.; Quinzi, V.; Mattei, A.; Marzo, G. Alcohol-free essential oils containing mouthrinse efficacy on three-day supragingival plaque regrowth: A randomized crossover clinical trial. *Trials* **2017**, *18*, 154. [CrossRef] [PubMed]
14. Arweiler, N.B.; Marx, V.K.; Laugisch, O.; Sculean, A.; Auschill, T.M. Clinical evaluation of a newly developed chairside test to determine periodontal pathogens. *J. Periodontol.* **2020**, *91*, 387–395. [CrossRef] [PubMed]
15. Bagavad Gita, J.; George, A.V.; Pavithra, N.; Chandrasekaran, S.C.; Latchumanadhas, K.; Gnanamani, A. Dysregulation of miR-146a by periodontal pathogens: A risk for acute coronary syndrome. *J. Periodontol.* **2019**, *90*, 756–765. [CrossRef]
16. Isola, G.; Alibrandi, A.; Curro, M.; Matarese, M.; Ricca, S.; Matarese, G.; Ientile, R.; Kocher, T. Evaluation of salivary and serum ADMA levels in patients with periodontal and cardiovascular disease as subclinical marker of cardiovascular risk. *J. Periodontol.* **2020**, *91*, 1076–1084. [CrossRef]
17. Mummolo, S.; Nota, A.; Albani, F.; Marchetti, E.; Gatto, R.; Marzo, G.; Quinzi, V.; Tecco, S. Salivary levels of Streptococcus mutans and Lactobacilli and other salivary indices in patients wearing clear aligners versus fixed orthodontic appliances: An observational study. *PLoS ONE* **2020**, *15*, e0228798. [CrossRef]
18. Vieira, A.R. Genetics of Periodontitis without Bias. *J. Periodontal. Res.* **2019**, *54*, 453–454. [CrossRef]
19. Li, G.; Robles, S.; Lu, Z.; Li, Y.; Krayer, J.W.; Leite, R.S.; Huang, Y. Upregulation of free fatty acid receptors in periodontal tissues of patients with metabolic syndrome and periodontitis. *J. Periodontal. Res.* **2019**, *54*, 356–363. [CrossRef]
20. Li, W.; Wang, X.; Tian, Y.; Xu, L.; Zhang, L.; Shi, D.; Feng, X.; Lu, R.; Meng, H. A novel multi-locus genetic risk score identifies patients with higher risk of generalized aggressive periodontitis. *J. Periodontol.* **2019**, *91*, 925–932. [CrossRef]
21. Isola, G. Current Evidence of Natural Agents in Oral and Periodontal Health. *Nutrients* **2020**, *12*. [CrossRef] [PubMed]
22. Isola, G.; Polizzi, A.; Iorio-Siciliano, V.; Alibrandi, A.; Ramaglia, L.; Leonardi, R. Effectiveness of a nutraceutical agent in the non-surgical periodontal therapy: A randomized, controlled clinical trial. *Clin. Oral Investig.* **2020**. [CrossRef]
23. Liu, Z.; Guo, H.; Zhang, W.; Ni, L. Salivary Microbiota Shifts under Sustained Consumption of Oolong Tea in Healthy Adults. *Nutrients* **2020**, *12*. [CrossRef] [PubMed]
24. Yan, K.; Lin, Q.; Tang, K.; Liu, S.; Du, Y.; Yu, X.; Li, S. Substance P participates in periodontitis by upregulating HIF-1alpha and RANKL/OPG ratio. *BMC Oral Health* **2020**, *20*, 27. [CrossRef] [PubMed]
25. Lee, J.H.; Park, Y.S.; Kim, Y.T.; Kim, D.H.; Jeong, S.N. Assessment of early discomfort and wound healing outcomes after periodontal surgery with and without enamel matrix derivative: An observational retrospective case-control study. *Clin. Oral Investig.* **2020**, *24*, 229–237. [CrossRef] [PubMed]
26. Cosgarea, R.; Tristiu, R.; Dumitru, R.B.; Arweiler, N.B.; Rednic, S.; Sirbu, C.I.; Lascu, L.; Sculean, A.; Eick, S. Effects of non-surgical periodontal therapy on periodontal laboratory and clinical data as well as on disease activity in patients with rheumatoid arthritis. *Clin. Oral Investig.* **2019**, *23*, 141–151. [CrossRef] [PubMed]
27. Wang, X.; Li, W.; Song, W.; Xu, L.; Zhang, L.; Feng, X.; Lu, R.; Meng, H. Association of CYP1A1 rs1048943 variant with aggressive periodontitis and its interaction with hyperlipidemia on the periodontal status. *J. Periodontal. Res.* **2019**, *54*, 546–554. [CrossRef] [PubMed]
28. Leonardi, R.; Loreto, C.; Talic, N.; Caltabiano, R.; Musumeci, G. Immunolocalization of lubricin in the rat periodontal ligament during experimental tooth movement. *Acta. Histochem.* **2012**, *114*, 700–704. [CrossRef]
29. Leonardi, R.; Almeida, L.E.; Trevilatto, P.C.; Loreto, C. Occurrence and regional distribution of TRAIL and DR5 on temporomandibular joint discs: Comparison of disc derangement with and without reduction. *Oral Surg. Oral Med. Oral Pathol. Oral Radiol. Endod.* **2010**, *109*, 244–251. [CrossRef]
30. Musumeci, G.; Trovato, F.M.; Loreto, C.; Leonardi, R.; Szychlinska, M.A.; Castorina, S.; Mobasheri, A. Lubricin expression in human osteoarthritic knee meniscus and synovial fluid: A morphological, immunohistochemical and biochemical study. *Acta Histochem* **2014**, *116*, 965–972. [CrossRef]
31. Mercuri, E.; Cassetta, M.; Cavallini, C.; Vicari, D.; Leonardi, R.; Barbato, E. Dental anomalies and clinical features in patients with maxillary canine impaction. *Angle Orthod.* **2013**, *83*, 22–28. [CrossRef] [PubMed]
32. Leonardi, R.; Farella, M.; Cobourne, M.T. An association between sella turcica bridging and dental transposition. *Eur. J. Orthod.* **2011**, *33*, 461–465. [CrossRef] [PubMed]

33. de, J.H.M.C.; Villafuerte, K.R.V.; Luchiari, H.R.; de, O.C.J.; Sales, M.; Palioto, D.B.; Messora, M.R.; Souza, S.L.S.; Taba, M., Jr.; Ramos, E.S.; et al. Effect of smoking on the DNA methylation pattern of the SOCS1 promoter in epithelial cells from the saliva of patients with chronic periodontitis. *J. Periodontol.* **2019**, *90*, 1279–1286. [CrossRef]
34. Taiete, T.; Casati, M.Z.; Martins, L.; Andia, D.C.; Mofatto, L.S.; Coletta, R.D.; Monteiro, M.F.; Araujo, C.F.; Santamaria, M.P.; Correa, M.G.; et al. Novel rare frameshift variation in aggressive periodontitis: Exomic and familial-screening analysis. *J. Periodontol.* **2020**, *91*, 263–273. [CrossRef] [PubMed]
35. Mijailovic, I.; Nikolic, N.; Djinic, A.; Carkic, J.; Milinkovic, I.; Peric, M.; Jankovic, S.; Milasin, J.; Aleksic, Z. The down-regulation of Notch 1 signaling contributes to the severity of bone loss in aggressive periodontitis. *J. Periodontol.* **2020**, *91*, 554–561. [CrossRef] [PubMed]
36. Briguglio, F.; Zenobio, E.G.; Isola, G.; Briguglio, R.; Briguglio, E.; Farronato, D.; Shibli, J.A. Complications in surgical removal of impacted mandibular third molars in relation to flap design: Clinical and statistical evaluations. *Quintessence Int.* **2011**, *42*, 445–453.
37. Jekabsone, A.; Sile, I.; Cochis, A.; Makrecka-Kuka, M.; Laucaityte, G.; Makarova, E.; Rimondini, L.; Bernotiene, R.; Raudone, L.; Vedlugaite, E.; et al. Investigation of Antibacterial and Antiinflammatory Activities of Proanthocyanidins from Pelargonium sidoides DC Root Extract. *Nutrients* **2019**, *11*. [CrossRef]
38. Lo Giudice, A.; Ortensi, L.; Farronato, M.; Lucchese, A.; Lo Castro, E.; Isola, G. The step further smile virtual planning: Milled versus prototyped mock-ups for the evaluation of the designed smile characteristics. *BMC Oral Health* **2020**, *20*, 165. [CrossRef]
39. Daniele, V.; Macera, L.; Taglieri, G.; Di Giambattista, A.; Spagnoli, G.; Massaria, A.; Messori, M.; Quagliarini, E.; Chiappini, G.; Campanella, V.; et al. Thermoplastic Disks Used for Commercial Orthodontic Aligners: Complete Physicochemical and Mechanical Characterization. *Materials* **2020**, *13*. [CrossRef]
40. Saccomanno, S.; Quinzi, V.; Sarhan, S.; Lagana, D.; Marzo, G. Perspectives of tele-orthodontics in the COVID-19 emergency and as a future tool in daily practice. *Eur. J. Paediatr. Dent.* **2020**, *21*, 157–162. [CrossRef]
41. Rosa, M., Quinzi, V., Marzo, G. Paediatric Orthodontics Part 1: Anterior open bite in the mixed dentition *Eur. J. Paediatr. Dent.* **2019**, *20*, 80–82. [CrossRef] [PubMed]
42. Lo Giudice, A.; Quinzi, V.; Ronsivalle, V.; Farronato, M.; Nicotra, C.; Indelicato, F.; Isola, G. Evaluation of Imaging Software Accuracy for 3-Dimensional Analysis of the Mandibular Condyle. A Comparative Study Using a Surface-to-Surface Matching Technique. *Int. J. Environ. Res. Public Health* **2020**, *17*. [CrossRef]
43. Lo Giudice, A.; Leonardi, R.; Ronsivalle, V.; Allegrini, S.; Lagravère, M.; Marzo, G.; Isola, G. Evaluation of pulp cavity/chamber changes after tooth-borne and bone-borne rapid maxillary expansion. A CBCT study using surface-based superimposition and deviation analysis. *Clin. Oral Investig.* **2020**. [CrossRef] [PubMed]
44. Lo Giudice, A.; Caccianiga, G.; Crimi, S.; Cavallini, C.; Leonardi, R. Frequency and type of ponticulus posticus in a longitudinal sample of nonorthodontically treated patients: Relationship with gender, age, skeletal maturity, and skeletal malocclusion. *Oral Surg. Oral Med. Oral Pathol. Oral Radiol.* **2018**, *126*, 291–297. [CrossRef] [PubMed]
45. Lo Giudice, A.; Nucera, R.; Perillo, L.; Paiusco, A.; Caccianiga, G. Is Low-Level Laser Therapy an Effective Method to Alleviate Pain Induced by Active Orthodontic Alignment Archwire? A Randomized Clinical Trial. *J. Evid. Based Dent. Pract.* **2019**, *19*, 71–78. [CrossRef]
46. Lo Giudice, A.; Rustico, L.; Caprioglio, A.; Migliorati, M.; Nucera, R. Evaluation of condylar cortical bone thickness in patient groups with different vertical facial dimensions using cone-beam computed tomography. *Odontology* **2020**, *108*, 669–675. [CrossRef]
47. Lo Giudice, A.; Spinuzza, P.; Rustico, L.; Messina, G.; Nucera, R. Short-term treatment effects produced by rapid maxillary expansion evaluated with computer tomography: A systematic review with meta-analysis. *The Korean J. Orthod.* **2020**, *37*. [CrossRef]
48. Perillo, L.; Padricelli, G.; Isola, G.; Femiano, F.; Chiodini, P.; Matarese, G. Class II malocclusion division 1: A new classification method by cephalometric analysis. *Eur. J. Paediatr. Dent.* **2012**, *13*, 192–196.
49. Marra, P.; Nucci, L.; Abdolreza, J.; Perillo, L.; Itro, A.; Grassia, V. Odontoma in a young and anxious patient associated with unerupted permanent mandibular cuspid: A case report. *J. Int. Oral Health* **2020**, *12*, 182–186. [CrossRef]

50. Cozzani, M.; Nucci, L.; Lupini, D.; Dolatshahizand, H.; Fazeli, D.; Barzkar, E.; Naeini, E.; Jamilian, A. The ideal insertion angle after immediate loading in Jeil, Storm, and Thunder miniscrews: A 3D-FEM study. *Int. Orthod.* **2020**, *18*, 503–508. [CrossRef]
51. Cozzani, M.; Sadri, D.; Nucci, L.; Jamilian, P.; Pirhadirad, A.P.; Jamilian, A. The effect of Alexander, Gianelly, Roth, and MBT bracket systems on anterior retraction: A 3-dimensional finite element study. *Clin. Oral Investig.* **2020**, *24*, 1351–1357. [CrossRef] [PubMed]
52. Shinjo, T.; Ishikado, A.; Hasturk, H.; Pober, D.M.; Paniagua, S.M.; Shah, H.; Wu, I.H.; Tinsley, L.J.; Matsumoto, M.; Keenan, H.A.; et al. Characterization of periodontitis in people with type 1 diabetes of 50 years or longer duration. *J. Periodontol.* **2019**, *90*, 565–575. [CrossRef] [PubMed]
53. Morelli, T.; Moss, K.L.; Preisser, J.S.; Beck, J.D.; Divaris, K.; Wu, D.; Offenbacher, S. Periodontal profile classes predict periodontal disease progression and tooth loss. *J. Periodontol.* **2018**, *89*, 148–156. [CrossRef]
54. Bogdan, M.; Meca, A.D.; Boldeanu, M.V.; Gheorghe, D.N.; Turcu-Stiolica, A.; Subtirelu, M.S.; Boldeanu, L.; Blaj, M.; Botnariu, G.E.; Vlad, C.E.; et al. Possible Involvement of Vitamin C in Periodontal Disease-Diabetes Mellitus Association. *Nutrients* **2020**, *12*. [CrossRef] [PubMed]
55. Nastri, L.; Moretti, A.; Migliaccio, S.; Paoletta, M.; Annunziata, M.; Liguori, S.; Toro, G.; Bianco, M.; Cecoro, G.; Guida, L.; et al. Do Dietary Supplements and Nutraceuticals Have Effects on Dental Implant Osseointegration? A Scoping Review. *Nutrients* **2020**, *12*. [CrossRef] [PubMed]

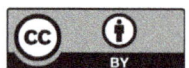

© 2020 by the author. Licensee MDPI, Basel, Switzerland. This article is an open access article distributed under the terms and conditions of the Creative Commons Attribution (CC BY) license (http://creativecommons.org/licenses/by/4.0/).

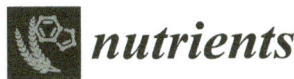

Editorial

Current Evidence of Natural Agents in Oral and Periodontal Health

Gaetano Isola

Department of General Surgery and Surgical-Medical Specialties, Unit of Oral Surgery and Periodontology, School of Dentistry, University of Catania, Via S. Sofia 78, 95124 Catania, Italy; gaetano.isola@unict.it

Received: 30 January 2020; Accepted: 12 February 2020; Published: 24 February 2020

Abstract: Oral and periodontal diseases, chewing disorders, and many destructive inflammatory diseases of the supporting tissues of the teeth are usually caused by an imbalance between host defense and environmental factors like smoking, poor nutrition, and a high percentage of periodontopathogenic bacteria. For these reasons, it is important also to focus attention on plaque control and also on improving host resistance through smoking and stress reduction, and a healthy diet. During the last decades, the importance of micronutrients has been extensively reviewed, and it was concluded that the prevention and treatment of periodontitis should include correct daily nutrition and a correct balance between antioxidants, probiotics, natural agents, vitamin D, and calcium. Recently, there has been growing interest in the literature on the impact of nutraceutical dietary aliments on oral and general health. This Special Issue provides a current and thoughtful perspective on the relationship of diet and natural agents on oral and periodontal diseases through a correct clinical approach with the last and most important evidence that may determine good oral conditions and high quality of life.

Keywords: periodontitis; natural agents; gingivitis; antioxidants; vitamins

---

It has been widely demonstrated that herbal medicines, which include medicinal herbs, herbal preparations, and phytotherapeutic compounds (that have plant or natural materials), have real therapeutic benefits for humans [1–3]. Worldwide, about 80% of the population uses phytotherapeutic products such as extracts, vitamins, tea, and other similar principles for various reasons for the treatment of various pathologies, with a cost of over 50 billion dollars a year in the global market [4]. This high consumption of herbal products compared to traditional drugs, such as antibiotics, is attributable to the large margin of safety and tolerability of natural agents, which could lead to a possible reduction in the long-term on the total national economic costs compared to traditional drugs. In addition, conventional drugs have also been shown to have a higher incidence of side effects, allergies, and resistance, especially antibiotics [5,6]. Therefore, herbal medicines are increasingly being used both as food supplements and to prevent or treat common oral and systemic diseases [5].

Among the main diseases of the stomatognathic apparatus, periodontitis is a chronic inflammatory disease caused by oral bacteria that determines the destruction of the supporting structures of the teeth [7–9]. The etiology of periodontitis is multifactorial with the bacteria of the oral biofilm which are fundamental for the initiation and progression of the disease. The different forms of periodontal disease are very different around the world but reach a total incidence rate of over 60%. The bacterial origin of periodontitis has been widely demonstrated, starting from an imbalance in aerobic and anaerobic biofilm bacteria [10], which can lead, under specific conditions, to activation of the host response, especially of neutrophilic bacteria and related products, which determines the disruption of soft and hard oral tissues [11–13]. This imbalance of the host response through the immune system results in further up or down-regulation of various pro-inflammatory cytokines, which finally determines the release of rapid oxidative stress (ROS) cells and neutrophil mediators [14,15]. This prolonged inflammatory status on the hard and soft tissues of the periodontium, including the connective tissue, leads to the degradation and consequent loss of the periodontal structure of the tooth and of the alveolar bone, causing, in the final disease steps, tooth loss [16].

Several studies have shown, in damaged periodontal tissues, a direct association between increased levels of inflammatory mediators induced by reactive oxygen species (such as NO) and the worsening of periodontitis [17,18]. Therefore, herbal medicines have been demonstrated to have an important role due to their broad spectrum of action against ROS and NO mediators, together with a good safety and tolerability margin compared with traditional drugs in both children and adults [19–23].

A good adjuvant response in both surgical and nonsurgical periodontal treatment has been shown in recent years by natural agents. Especially in the non-surgical approach, various antimicrobials and chemotherapy agents, including chlorhexidine, triclosan, desiccant agents, vitamin and probiotic compounds, and cetylpyridinium chloride, have been studied and validated for the management of periodontitis [24–29]. However, even more studies have aimed at analyzing phytotherapeutic drugs in order to obtain antimicrobial, antiseptic, anti-inflammatory, and antioxidant effects during periodontitis.

In fact, herbal medicines have been shown to possess a wide and specific range of biological properties including antimicrobial, antioxidant and anti-inflammatory effects at the oral and systemic levels. The natural phytotherapeutic compounds, including medicinal herbs, help to suppress the inflammatory response, which determines, in the long term, the destruction of the hard and soft tissues of the oral cavity, characteristic in various oral diseases, including periodontitis [30–34]. Among the main anti-inflammatory actions due to phytotherapy drugs, there is, above all, an anti-inflammatory and oxidative action which leads to excellent therapeutic action in the long-term. However, on the other hand, various studies in the oral field that have analyzed the actions of traditional and phytotherapeutic drugs have given uncertain results that require large-scale populations to be validated [35–39].

Based on these findings, the aim of this Special Issue is to further analyze the therapeutic effects of these medicinal herbs, phytotherapy, and of the main inflammatory mediator characteristics of oral and periodontal diseases.

Given the many new aspects related to the optimal management of phytotherapy drugs in dentistry, it was my pleasure to receive publications detailing the results of different joint research groups for this highly stimulating Special Issue on this subject that is aimed at analyzing and validating new scientific approaches to improve the prevention and treatment of oral and periodontal diseases through the use of phytotherapeutic drugs.

Author Contributions: Conceptualization, writing—original draft preparation, G.I.; G.I. has read and agreed to the published version of the manuscript.

Funding: This research received no external funding.

Conflicts of Interest: The author declares no conflict of interest.

References

1. Tambekar, D.H.; Dahikar, S.B.; Lahare, M.D. Antibacterial potentials of some herbal preparations available in India. *Res. J. Med. Med. Sci.* **2009**, *4*, 224–227.
2. Mohammed, H.; Varoni, E.M.; Cochis, A.; Cordaro, M.; Gallenzi, P.; Patini, R.; Staderini, E.; Lajolo, C.; Rimondini, L.; Rocchetti, V. Oral dysbiosis in pancreatic cancer and liver cirrhosis: A review of the literature. *Biomedicines* **2018**, *4*, 115. [CrossRef] [PubMed]
3. Patini, R.; Gallenzi, P.; Spagnuolo, G.; Cordaro, M.; Cantiani, M.; Amalfitano, A.; Arcovito, A.; Callà, C.A.M.; Mingrone, G.; Nocca, G. Correlation between metabolic syndrome, periodontitis and reactive oxygen species production. A pilot study. *Open Dent. J.* **2017**, *11*, 621–627. [CrossRef]
4. World Health Organization. The World Medicines Situation 2011. In *Traditional Medicines: Global Situation, Issues and Challenges*; WHO: Geneva, Switzerland, 2011; pp. 1–14.
5. Wu, Y.H.; Kuraji, R.; Taya, Y.; Ito, H.; Numabe, Y. Effects of theaflavins on tissue inflammation and bone resorption on experimental periodontitis in rats. *J. Periodontal Res.* **2018**, *53*, 1009–1019. [CrossRef] [PubMed]

6. Isola, G.; Polizzi, A.; Santonocito, S.; Alibrandi, A.; Ferlito, S. Expression of Salivary And Serum Malondialdehyde And Lipid Profile Of Patients With Periodontitis And Coronary Heart Disease. *Int. J. Mol. Sci.* **2019**, *20*, 6061. [CrossRef] [PubMed]
7. Isola, G.; Matarese, G.; Ramaglia, L.; Pedullà, E.; Rapisarda, E.; Iorio-Siciliano, V. Association between periodontitis and glycosylated haemoglobin before diabetes onset: A cross-sectional study. *Clin. Oral Investig.* **2019**. [CrossRef] [PubMed]
8. Patini, R.; Staderini, E.; Gallenzi, P. Multidisciplinary surgical management of Cowden syndrome: Report of a case. *J. Clin. Exp. Dent.* **2016**, *8*, e472. [CrossRef]
9. Facciolo, M.T.; Riva, F.; Gallenzi, P.; Patini, R.; Gaglioti, D. A rare case of oral multisystem Langerhans cell histiocytosis. *J. Clin. Exp. Dent.* **2017**, *9*, e820. [CrossRef]
10. Nilsson, H.; Berglund, J.S.; Renvert, S. Periodontitis, tooth loss and cognitive functions among older adults. *Clin. Oral Investig.* **2018**, *22*, 2103–2109. [CrossRef]
11. Isola, G.; Anastasi, G.; Matarese, G.; Williams, R.C.; Cutroneo, G.; Bracco, P.; Piancino, M.G. Functional and molecular outcomes of the human masticatory muscles. *Oral Dis.* **2018**, *8*, 1424–1441. [CrossRef]
12. Isola, G.; Polizzi, A.; Alibrandi, A.; Indelicato, F.; Ferlito, S. Analysis of Endothelin-1 concentrations in individuals with periodontitis. *Sci. Rep.* **2020**, *10*, 1652. [CrossRef]
13. Staderini, E.; Patini, R.; de Luca, M.; Gallenzi, P. Three-dimensional stereophotogrammetric analysis of nasolabial soft tissue effects of rapid maxillary expansion: A systematic review of clinical trials. *Acta Otorhinolaryngol. Ital.* **2018**, *38*, 399–408. [PubMed]
14. Isola, G.; Perillo, L.; Migliorati, M.; Matarese, M.; Dalessandri, D.; Grassia, V.; Alibrandi, A.; Matarese, G. The impact of temporomandibular joint arthritis on functional disability and global health in patients with juvenile idiopathic arthritis. *Eur. J. Orthod.* **2019**, *41*, 117–124. [CrossRef] [PubMed]
15. Isola, G.; Alibrandi, A.; Rapisarda, E.; Matarese, G.; Williams, R.C.; Leonardi, R. Association of Vitamin d in patients with periodontitis: A cross-sectional study. *J. Periodontal Res.* **2020**. In Press.
16. Nadelman, P.; Magno, M.B.; Masterson, D.; da Cruz, A.G.; Maia, L.C. Are dairy products containing probiotics beneficial for oral health? A systematic review and meta-analysis. *Clin. Oral Investig.* **2018**, *22*, 2763–2785. [CrossRef] [PubMed]
17. Isola, G.; Lo Giudice, A.; Polizzi, A.; Alibrandi, A.; Patini, R.; Ferlito, S. Periodontitis and Tooth Loss Have Negative Systemic Impact on Circulating Progenitor Cell Levels: A Clinical Study. *Genes* **2019**, *10*, 1022. [CrossRef]
18. Pippi, R.; Santoro, M.; Patini, R. The central odontogenic fibroma: How difficult can be making a preliminary diagnosis. *J. Clin. Exp. Dent.* **2016**, *8*, e223–e225. [CrossRef]
19. Grassia, V.; D'Apuzzo, F.; Ferrulli, V.E.; Matarese, G.; Femiano, F.; Perillo, L. Dento-skeletal effects of mixed palatal expansion evaluated by postero-anterior cephalometric analysis. *Eur. J. Paediatr Dent.* **2014**, *15*, 59–62.
20. Grassia, V.; D'Apuzzo, F.; Di Stasio, D.; Jamilian, A.; Lucchese, A.; Perillo, L. Upper and lower arch changes after Mixed Palatal Expansion protocol. *Eur. J. Paediatr Dent.* **2014**, *15*, 375–380.
21. Moura, M.F.; Navarro, T.P.; Silva, T.A.; Cota, L.O.M. Soares Dutra Oliveira AM, Costa FO. Periodontitis and Endothelial Dysfunction: Periodontal Clinical Parameters and Levels of Salivary Markers Interleukin-1β, Tumor Necrosis Factor-α, Matrix Metalloproteinase-2, Tissue Inhibitor of Metalloproteinases-2 Complex, and Nitric Oxide. *J. Periodontol.* **2017**, *88*, 778–787.
22. Coviello, V.; Zareh Dehkhargani, S.; Patini, R.; Cicconetti, A. Surgical ciliated cyst 12 years after Le Fort I maxillary advancement osteotomy: A case report and review of the literature. *Oral Surg.* **2017**, *10*, 165–170. [CrossRef]
23. Isola, G.; Matarese, M.; Ramaglia, L.; Iorio-Siciliano, V.; Cordasco, G.; Matarese, G. Efficacy of a drug composed of herbal extracts on postoperative discomfort after surgical removal of impacted mandibular third molar: A randomized, triple-blind, controlled clinical trial. *Clin. Oral Investig.* **2019**, *23*, 2443–2453. [CrossRef] [PubMed]
24. Grassia, V.; Lombardi, A.; Kawasaki, H.; Ferri, C.; Perillo, L.; Mosca, L.; Delle Cave, D.; Nucci, L.; Porcelli, M.; Caraglia, M. Salivary microRNAs as new molecular markers in cleft lip and palate: A new frontier in molecular medicine. *Oncotarget* **2018**, *9*, 18929–18930. [CrossRef] [PubMed]
25. Kırzıoğlu, F.Y.; Özmen, Ö.; Doğan, B.; Bulut, M.T.; Fentoğlu, Ö.; Özdem, M. Effects of rosuvastatin on inducible nitric oxide synthase in rats with hyperlipidaemia and periodontitis. *J. Periodontal Res.* **2018**, *53*, 258–266. [CrossRef]

26. Nastri, L.; de Rosa, A.; de Gregorio, V.; Grassia, V.; Donnarumma, G. A New Controlled-Release Material Containing Metronidazole and Doxycycline for the Treatment of Periodontal and Peri-Implant Diseases: Formulation and in Vitro Testing. *Int. J. Dent.* **2019**, *2019*, 9374607. [CrossRef]
27. Isola, G.; Polizzi, A.; Muraglie, S.; Leonardi, R.M.; Lo Giudice, A. Assessment of vitamin C and Antioxidants Profiles In Saliva and Serum in Patients With Periodontitis and Ischemic Heart Disease. *Nutrients* **2019**, *11*, 2956. [CrossRef]
28. Isola, G.; Alibrandi, A.; Currò, M.; Matarese, M.; Ricca, S.; Matarese, G.; Ientile, R.; Kocher, T. Evaluation of salivary and serum ADMA levels in patients with periodontal and cardiovascular disease as subclinical marker of cardiovascular risk. *J. Periodontol.* **2020**. [CrossRef]
29. Isola, G.; Matarese, M.; Ramaglia, L.; Cicciù, M.; Matarese, G. Evaluation of the efficacy of celecoxib and ibuprofen on postoperative pain, swelling, and mouth opening after surgical removal of impacted third molars: A randomized, controlled clinical trial. *Int. J. Oral Maxillofac. Surg.* **2019**, *48*, 1348–1354. [CrossRef]
30. Loreto, C.; Almeida, L.E.; Trevilatto, P.; Leonardi, R. Apoptosis in displaced temporomandibular joint disc with and without reduction: An immunohistochemical study. *J. Oral Pathol. Med.* **2011**, *40*, 103–110. [CrossRef]
31. Leonardi, R.; Lo Giudice, A.; Rugeri, M.; Muraglie, S.; Cordasco, G.; Barbato, E. Three-dimensional evaluation on digital casts of maxillary palatal size and morphology in patients with functional posterior crossbite. *Eur. J. Orthod.* **2018**, *40*, 556–562. [CrossRef]
32. Lo Giudice, A.; Nucera, R.; Perillo, L.; Paiusco, A.; Caccianiga, G. Is low-level laser therapy an effective method to alleviate pain induced by active orthodontic alignment archwire? A randomized clinical trial. *J. Evid. Based Dent. Pract.* **2019**, *19*, 71–78. [CrossRef] [PubMed]
33. Lo Giudice, A.; Barbato, E.; Cosentino, L.; Ferraro, C.M.; Leonardi, R. Alveolar bone changes after rapid maxillary expansion with tooth-born appliances: A systematic review. *Eur. J. Orthod.* **2018**, *40*, 296–303. [CrossRef] [PubMed]
34. Lo Giudice, A.; Caccianiga, G.; Crimi, S.; Cavallini, C.; Leonardi, R. Frequency and type of ponticulus posticus in a longitudinal sample of nonorthodontically treated patients: Relationship with gender, age, skeletal maturity, and skeletal malocclusion. *Oral. Surg. Oral. Med. Oral Pathol. Oral. Radiol.* **2018**, *126*, 291–297. [CrossRef] [PubMed]
35. Scalzone, A.; Flores-Mir, C.; Carozza, D.; D'Apuzzo, F.; Grassia, V.; Perillo, L. Secondary alveolar bone grafting using autologous versus alloplastic material in the treatment of cleft lip and palate patients: Systematic review and meta-analysis. *Prog. Orthod.* **2019**, *20*, 6. [CrossRef]
36. Piancino, M.G.; Isola, G.; Cannavale, R.; Cutroneo, G.; Vermiglio, G.; Bracco, P.; Anastasi, G.P. From periodontal mechanoreceptors to chewing motor control: A systematic review. *Arch. Oral Biol.* **2017**, *78*, 109–121. [CrossRef]
37. Zeidán-Chuliá, F.; Yilmaz, D.; Häkkinen, L.; Könönen, E.; Neves de Oliveira, B.H.; Güncü, G.; Uitto, V.J.; Caglayan, F.; Gürsoy, U.K. Matrix metalloproteinase-7 in periodontitis with type 2 diabetes mellitus. *J. Periodontal Res.* **2018**, *53*, 916–923. [CrossRef]
38. Cutroneo, G.; Piancino, M.G.; Ramieri, G.; Bracco, P.; Vita, G.; Isola, G.; Vermiglio, G.; Favaloro, A.; Anastasi, G.; Trimarchi, F. Expression of muscle-specific integrins in masseter muscle fibers during malocclusion disease. *Int. J. Mol. Med.* **2012**, *30*, 235–242. [CrossRef]
39. Scarel-Caminaga, R.M.; Cera, F.F.; Pigossi, S.C.; Finoti, L.S.; Kim, Y.J.; Viana, A.C.; Secolin, R.; Montenegro, M.F.; Tanus-Santos, J.E.; Orrico, S.R.P.; et al. Inducible Nitric Oxide Synthase Polymorphisms and Nitric Oxide Levels in Individuals with Chronic Periodontitis. *Int. J. Mol. Sci.* **2017**, *18*, 1128. [CrossRef]

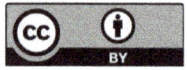

© 2020 by the author. Licensee MDPI, Basel, Switzerland. This article is an open access article distributed under the terms and conditions of the Creative Commons Attribution (CC BY) license (http://creativecommons.org/licenses/by/4.0/).

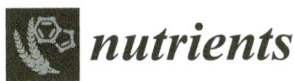

Article

Salivary Microbiota Shifts under Sustained Consumption of Oolong Tea in Healthy Adults

Zhibin Liu, Hongwen Guo, Wen Zhang and Li Ni *

Institute of Food Science & Technology, Fuzhou University, Fuzhou 350108, China; liuzhibin@fzu.edu.cn (Z.L.); guohongwen@fzu.edu.cn (H.G.); zhangwen@fzu.edu.cn (W.Z.)
* Correspondence: nili@fzu.edu.cn; Tel.: +86-591-2286-6378

Received: 16 February 2020; Accepted: 25 March 2020; Published: 31 March 2020

Abstract: Tea is the most widely consumed beverages next to water, however little is known about the influence of sustained tea consumption on the oral bacteria of healthy adults. In this study, three oral healthy adults were recruited and instructed to consume 1.0 L of oolong tea infusions (total polyphenol content, 2.83 g/L) daily, for eight weeks. Salivary microbiota pre-, peri-, and post-treatment were fully compared by high-throughput 16S rRNA sequencing and multivariate statistical analysis. It was revealed that oolong tea consumption reduced salivary bacterial diversity and the population of some oral disease related bacteria, such as *Streptococcus* sp., *Prevotella nanceiensis*, *Fusobacterium periodonticum*, *Alloprevotella rava*, and *Prevotella elaninogenica*. Moreover, via correlation network and Venn diagram analyses, seven bacterial taxa, including *Streptococcus* sp. (OTU_1), *Ruminococcaceae* sp. (OTU_33), *Haemophilus* sp. (OTU_696), *Veillonella* spp. (OTU_133 and OTU_23), *Actinomyces odontolyticus* (OTU_42), and *Gemella haemolysans* (OTU_6), were significantly altered after oolong tea consumption, and presented robust strong connections ($|r| > 0.9$ and $p < 0.05$) with other oral microbiota. These results suggest sustained oolong tea consumption would modulate salivary microbiota and generate potential oral pathogen preventative benefits. Additionally, diverse responses to oolong tea consumption among subjects were also noticed.

Keywords: oolong tea; phenolic profile; salivary microbiota; 16S rRNA sequencing; bacterial diversities; correlation network

1. Introduction

An estimation of 700 diverse bacterial species have been identified in human oral cavities, which constitute complex microbial communities [1]. These bacteria generally inhabit at different oral niches, including saliva, supragingival plaque, subgingival plaque, and mucosa. Of these niches, saliva harbors as much as 10^8 bacteria/mL and constitutes a reservoir of microorganisms regularly derived from dental plaque biofilms adhering to gingival crevices, periodontal pockets, the dorsum of the tongue, and other oral mucosal surfaces [2]. As an integral part of oral microbiota, salivary microbiota has been found to be differentiated between patients with a healthy oral cavity and those with dental caries and periodontitis [3]. Additionally, several studies discovered marked clinical importance of salivary microbiota on the general health of the host, such as by either preventing or causing infections [4]. Thus, salivary microbiota may provide further insight into the integral microbiota structure within the human oral cavity, and even the oral and general health status of individuals.

Since the oral cavity is exposed to the external environment, the salivary microbiota may be influenced by various factors, including oral hygiene, smoking, nutrients, mechanical stress, and the overall health condition of the host [5]. The impact of nutritional factors in shaping the oral microbial ecosystem cannot be ignored. Food residuals in the mouth can be utilized as substrates for oral bacteria; moreover, some food components have a selective effect on microbial growth, by either stimulating or suppressing some specific bacteria. For example, a regular consumption of polyphenol-rich beverages and foods, such as tea, cranberry, coffee, grape, almond, and alcohol-free red wine, have been reported to inhibit oral pathogenic bacteria [6–8]. The suppression of oral, especially periodontal pathogenic, bacteria may ameliorate the control of plaque biofilms, and thus reduce the inflammatory and immunological processes of oral and periodontal diseases [9]. Recently, the impact of nutraceutical dietary aliments, such as antioxidants, probiotics, natural agents, and vitamins, on oral health is gaining more and more attention [10].

Tea (*Camellia sinensis*), second only to water, is the most widely consumed beverage in the world. The major constituents of tea leaves are the flavonoids, including flavonols, flavones, and flavan-3-ols, of which over 60% are the flavan-3-ols, commonly referred to as catechins. Based on the United States Department of Agriculture (USDA) Flavonoid Database, it has been estimated that the daily total flavonoid intake is mainly from flavan-3-ols (83.5%); while, the major source of flavonoids is tea (157 mg), and citrus fruit juices come second (8 mg) [11]. There is a large population of heavy tea consumers all over the world, especially in the southern part of China, where people consume a substantial amount of tea infusions on a daily basis. A number of health-promoting effects have been associated with tea consumption; these effects are generally attributed to the phenolic compounds in tea. Tea polyphenols are well known for their antimicrobial properties, including on *Streptococcus mutans* and *lactobacilli* [12], and thus, they are believed to possess anti-cariogenic effects [13,14]. Moreover, regular consumption of tea has proved to exert gut microbiota regulation effect [15,16]. However, with regard to the normal balanced oral microbiota, little is known about the influence of tea drinking. Considering the wide range of biological properties, including anti-microbial, anti-oxidant, anti-inflammatory, anti-cariogenic, and gut microbiota regulation effects of tea polyphenols, it is reasonable to assume that sustained tea drinking will result in certain oral ecological shifts. A better understanding of the oral ecological shifts under sustained and significant tea consumption may contribute to oral health management for tea consumers.

It is also worth noting that, due to the variability in genes, social habits, hormonal fluctuation, diet, quality and quantity of saliva, etc., the oral environment differs between subjects and represents huge inter-individual variations [17]. Moreover, the responses of oral microbiota of different individuals to certain nutritional factors maybe also be diverse. To understand the influence of tea consumption on oral microbiota, tracking the temporal dynamic of salivary microbiota of subjects separately may provide useful information free from interference of inter-individual variations. In the current study, it is hypothesized that sustained tea consumption will alter the composition of salivary microbiota and exert oral health benefits to the host. To test this hypothesis, three orally healthy subjects were recruited and instructed to consume a substantial amount of tea infusions on a daily basis and their salivary bacterial communities pre-, peri-, and post-treatment were quantified by utilizing a high-throughput HiSeq sequencing technique. Then, via several multivariate statistical analyses, the temporal dynamics of salivary microbiota of each individual were analyzed. Based on these, the impact of sustained consumption of tea on the normal balanced oral microbiota was discussed.

2. Materials and Methods

2.1. Oolong Tea Infusion Preparation and Phenolic Profile Analysis

The tea used in this study was an oolong tea variety, purchased from a local market in Fujian Province, China. The oolong tea was prepared in accordance with the tea consumption method of local residents. A certain amount of dry oolong tea (whole leaves) was immersed in 20 times the volume of distilled boiling water (temperature around 90–95 °C) for 1 min, then the tea leaves were filtered, and the liquor was retained as an oolong tea infusion.

The phenolic profile of the tea infusion was then analyzed by utilizing ultra-high performance liquid chromatography (UHPLC) coupled to quadrupole time-of-flight mass spectrometer (Q-TOF MS/MS) approach, as previously described [15]. Briefly, chromatography separation was performed on an Acquity UHPLC system (Waters, Milford, MA, USA) with HSS T3 column (100 mm × 2.1 mm,

1.7 µm). A sample of 1 µL was injected and eluted with the mobile phase at 0.3 mL/min at 40 °C; detection was at 280 nm. The mobile phase consisted of (A) 0.1% formic acid solution (v/v) and (B) acetonitrile with 0.1% formic acid (v/v), while the gradient program was as follows: 99%–93% (A) in 0–2 min; 93%–60% (A) in 2–13 min; 60%–1% (A) in 13–14 min. The eluent was then introduced to a SYNAPT G2-Si high-definition mass spectrometer (Waters, Milford, MA, USA) equipped with an electrospray ionization (ESI) source. The analyses were performed in negative-ion mode and positive-ion mode, with a sampling cone voltage of 40.0 V, and a capillary voltage of 2500 V. The source temperature was 120 °C, with a desolvation gas flow of 800 L/h at a temperature of 450 °C. The time-of-flight (TOF) acquisition rate was 0.2 s/scan with 0.01 s inter-scan delay. Data were collected in centroid mode from 100 to 1200 Da in full scan during 0–14 min. The mass data were corrected during acquisition using a lock-mass calibrant of leucine enkephalin (200 ng/mL), via a lock spray interface at a flow-rate of 50 µL/min, generating a reference ion for positive ion mode ($[M+H]^+$ = 556.2771) and negative ion mode ($[M-H]^-$ = 554.2615) to ensure accuracy during the MS analysis. All data analyses were conducted using the MarkerLynx application manager software (version 4.1, Waters, Milford, MA, USA). The total polyphenols content in the tea infusions was then measured by utilizing the Folin–Ciocalteu method [18]. Briefly, 1 mL sample, 5 mL Folin–Ciocalteu's reagent (diluted 10 times), and 4 mL sodium carbonate (7.5%, w/v) were mixed. After 60 min, the absorbance at 765 nm was measured. Total phenolic content was expressed as a mass percentage on dry matter basis. Gallic acid was used as an external standard.

2.2. Subject Enrollment, Study Design, and Salivary Sample Collection

The inclusion criteria for this study included: healthy adult individuals sharing a relatively similar living environment; no tea and antibiotics taken in the previous 3 months; and no smoking. After the screening process, three healthy adult Chinese individuals (2 females and 1 male), 23 years of age, were enrolled from the campus of Fuzhou University, Fuzhou, China. The plaque and gingival status was examined before and after tea intervention. No obvious change was observed either before or after tea usage. In addition, no adverse reaction was reported throughout the experimental period by participants. Written informed consent was obtained from each participant. This study was approved by the ethical committee of the Institute of Food Science and Technology of Fuzhou University (approval number: IFSTFZU20180301).

This study consisted of a 3-day baseline period, an 8-week oolong tea infusion intervention period, and a 4-week follow-up period. During the intervention period, the three subjects (subject 1, subject 2, and subject 3) were required to consume 1.0 L of oolong tea infusion per day (0.5 L in the morning and 0.5 L in the afternoon). Moreover, they were also instructed to circulate or swish the infusion around in their mouths prior to swallowing the tea infusion. During the follow-up period, the subjects were asked not to consume any tea drinks. In addition to this, the subjects were asked to maintain their regular diet and oral hygiene habits, with the exception of the sampling occasions. Salivary samples were collected at 4 different stages, each stage included 3 sequential days: (A) 3 sequential days of the baseline period, which was prior to the intervention period; (B) 3 sequential days after 4 weeks of the tea intervention; (C) 3 sequential days after 8 weeks of the tea intervention; and (D) 3 sequential days at the end of the follow-up period, which accounted for 4 weeks post-intervention. All salivary sample collections were conducted in the morning. Each subject was asked not to eat, drink, or brush their teeth before the sample collection. Then, 2 mL of unstimulated saliva were collected from the subjects by expectoration into a tube. In total, 36 salivary samples from the 3 subjects were sampled.

2.3. Salivary Bacterial DNA Extraction

Salivary bacterial DNA was extracted from the 36 salivary samples by utilizing a rapid DNA extraction kit (BioTeke Corporation, Beijing, China), following the manufacturer's instructions. The extracted bacterial DNA was then checked by agarose gel electrophoresis.

2.4. Illumina Sequencing of Salivary Bacteria

Bacterial primers 341-F (5′-CCT AYG GGR BGC ASC AG-3′) and 806-R (5′-GGA CTA CNN GGG TAT CTA AT-3′) with specific barcodes were used to amplify the V3–V4 region of bacterial 16S rRNA genes. The sequencing library of bacterial 16S rRNA genes was generated for high-throughput sequencing, employing the TruSeq® DNA PCR-Free Sample Preparation Kit (Illumina, San Diego, CA, USA). Next, the library was sequenced on an Illumina HiSeq2500 platform by Novogene Bioinformatics Technology Co., Ltd. (Beijing, China).

2.5. Bioinformatic Analysis

Raw sequencing reads, obtained from the Illumina platform, were then merged by using FLASH software (Version 1.2.7) [19] and filtered using QIIME software (Version 1.7), with the default parameter setting of 'split_libraries_fastq.py' script [20,21]. All quality filtered sequencing reads were then clustered into operational taxonomic units (OTUs) with a threshold of 97% sequence similarity, by utilizing UPARSE software (Version 7.0) [22]. The representative sequence (most abundant) for each bacterial OTU was then annotated by utilizing the GreenGene Database [23] and Human Oral Microbiome Database (HOMD) [24]. The least total sequences number was 30,070 in this study. The total reads of each sample was normalized to 30,070 sequences/sample, and the OTUs abundance information was normalized correspondingly for further analysis.

Based on these annotated and normalized output data, different statistical methods were used to interpret the similarities of diverse data sets, or to plot the correlation network among the salivary microbiota. First, community diversity estimators including Shannon and Simpson indexes were calculated by R software (Version 3.2.5) with vegan package. Second, the multiple response permutation procedure (MRPP) and analysis of similarity (Anosim) were employed to compare the statistical differences within and between subjects in salivary microbiota profiles, by using R software with vegan package [23]. Third, principal component analysis (PCA) was applied to evaluate and visualize the differences of samples in OTU-level complexity, by using R software with mixOmics package. Next, the correlations among the OTUs with relative abundance over 0.1% of each subject were calculated, based upon Pearson's correlation coefficients, by using R software with Hmisc package. The strong connections ($|r| > 0.9$, $p < 0.05$) were further imported into Gephi software (Version 0.8.2), so as to generate correlation networks of these predominant microbiota [25]. The nodes (OTUs) with high strong connection numbers were defined as the "hub microbiota", which were likely to be more connected to other nodes when compared to non-hub nodes [26,27]. Moreover, the relative abundance of the hub microbiota was further visualized into heatmaps, by utilizing R software with pheatmap package. Hierarchical clustering of the columns (samples) was further calculated based on Euclidean distance and ward.D method, and indicated on the heatmaps. Lastly, in order to identify the shared and unique hub salivary microbiome of these three subjects, a Venn diagram was built according to the method as descripted by Heberle et al. [28].

Other data are expressed as mean ± SD. Furthermore, the statistical significance among different data sets was analyzed by Student's t-test or Duncan's multiple range test using SPSS software (Version 19.0.0), while the significance threshold was established at 0.05.

3. Results

3.1. Phenolic Profile of Oolong Tea Infusion

The total polyphenols content and phenolic profile of the oolong tea infusion used in this study were determined, and the results indicated that the total polyphenol content of the tea infusion was 2.83 ± 0.02 g/L. Following untargeted UHPLC Q-TOF-MS approach, the phenolic constituents present in the tea infusion were further analyzed. Table 1 gives the MS characteristics and tentative identification of each chromatographic peak. These chromatographic peaks, along with their proposed chemical structure, are depicted in Figure S1. In summary, 33 constituents were tentatively identified from the tea infusion, including 2 alkaloids, 7 flavan-3-ols, 7 organic acids and esters, 4 proanthocyanidins, 11 flavonoid glycosides, 1 theaflavin, and 1 amino acid. Of the total chromatographic peak areas, caffeine (peak 16), epigallocatechin (peak 13), epicatechin (peak 20), gallic acid (peak 5), and caffeoyl-hexoside (peak 1) were the most abundant constituents.

Table 1. The phenolic profiles of the oolong tea infusion.

Peak No. [a]	t_R (Min)	Tentative Identification	Chemical Formula	[M-H]$^-$ (m/z)		
				Measured Mass (Da)	Theoretical Exact Mass (Da)	Mass Accuracy (ppm)
1	1.05	Caffeoyl-hexoside	$C_{15}H_{18}O_9$	341.0875	341.0873	0.58
2	1.40	L-Theanine	$C_7H_{14}N_2O_3$	173.0931	173.0927	2.53
3	1.97	Epigallocatechin-glucuronide	$C_{21}H_{22}O_{13}$	481.0991	481.0983	1.74
4	2.49	Theasinensin C	$C_{30}H_{26}O_{14}$	609.1235	609.1245	−1.60
5	2.74	Gallic acid	$C_7H_6O_5$	169.0140	169.0137	1.52
6	2.92	Theogallin	$C_{14}H_{16}O_{10}$	343.0665	343.0666	−0.19
7	3.80	Theobromine [b]	$C_7H_8N_4O_2$	181.0736	181.0725	6.04
8	3.84	Gallocatechin	$C_{15}H_{14}O_7$	305.0662	305.0662	0.09
9	4.37	Theasinensin B	$C_{37}H_{30}O_{18}$	761.1348	761.1354	−0.83
10	4.41	Digalloyl-hexoside	$C_{20}H_{20}O_{14}$	483.0758	483.0775	−3.57
11	4.54	O-Methylgallic acid	$C_8H_8O_5$	183.0295	183.0294	0.58
12	4.81	Theacitrin A	$C_{37}H_{28}O_{18}$	759.1196	759.1198	−0.24
13	4.91	Epigallocatechin	$C_{15}H_{14}O_7$	305.0689	305.0662	8.94
14	5.16	p-Coumaroylquinic acid	$C_{16}H_{18}O_8$	337.0923	337.0924	−0.26
15	5.36	Catechin	$C_{15}H_{14}O_6$	289.0718	289.0713	1.87
16	5.60	Caffeine [b]	$C_8H_{10}N_4O_2$	195.0888	195.0882	3.30
17	5.68	Procyanidin	$C_{30}H_{26}O_{12}$	577.1356	577.1346	1.65
18	5.79	Epicatechin-epicatechin	$C_{30}H_{26}O_{12}$	577.1356	577.1346	1.65
19	6.14	p-Coumaroylquinic acid	$C_{16}H_{18}O_8$	337.0923	337.0924	−0.26
20	6.23	Epicatechin	$C_{15}H_{14}O_6$	289.0734	289.0713	7.41
21	6.34	Epigallocatechin gallate	$C_{22}H_{18}O_{11}$	457.0777	457.0771	1.24
22	6.41	p-Coumaroylquinic acid	$C_{16}H_{18}O_8$	337.0918	337.0924	−1.74
23	6.68	Gallocatechin gallate	$C_{22}H_{18}O_{11}$	457.0773	457.0771	0.37
24	6.92	Theaflavin	$C_{29}H_{24}O_{12}$	563.1199	563.1190	1.60
25	7.01	Myricetin hexoside	$C_{21}H_{20}O_{13}$	479.0827	479.0826	0.19
26	7.11	Myricetin-hexoside	$C_{21}H_{20}O_{13}$	479.0825	479.0826	−0.23
27	7.21	Quercetin-hexosyl-hexosyl-deoxyhexoside	$C_{33}H_{40}O_{21}$	771.1986	771.1984	0.22
28	7.36	Quercetin-hexosyl-hexosyl-deoxyhexoside	$C_{33}H_{40}O_{21}$	771.1982	771.1984	−0.30
29	7.62	Kaempferol-deoxyhexosyl-deoxyhexoside	$C_{27}H_{30}O_{14}$	577.1555	577.1558	−0.48
30	7.72	Kaempferol-hexosyl-hexosyl-deoxyhexoside	$C_{33}H_{40}O_{20}$	755.2029	755.2035	−0.81
31	8.00	Kaempferol-hexosyl-hexosyl-deoxyhexoside	$C_{33}H_{40}O_{20}$	755.2048	755.2035	1.70
32	8.43	Kaempferol-hexosyl-hexoside	$C_{27}H_{30}O_{15}$	593.1508	593.1507	0.18
33	8.78	Kaempferol-hexoside	$C_{21}H_{20}O_{11}$	447.0927	447.0928	−0.18

[a] Peaks were assigned from the chromatograms in Figure S1; [b] [M+H]$^+$ mode.

3.2. Overall Salivary Bacterial Structure

The salivary bacterial components of the three subjects during the 12-week experimental period were investigated and evaluated using the Illumina HiSeq sequencing analysis. A total of 1,983,489 (average length = 425 bp) quality filtered sequencing reads corresponding to the V3–V4 region of bacterial 16S rRNA genes were obtained. Good's coverage estimation values were within the range of 99.8%–100%, which indicated adequate sequence coverage to reliably describe the full bacterial communities present in all the samples. All sequences were clustered into 189 to 458 OTUs with a 97% similarity level for each sample. The summary of the sequencing results is listed in Table S1.

After the taxonomic assignment, these sequences were then annotated into 25 phyla and 260 genera. At the phylum level, *Firmicutes* (41.04%), *Bacteroidetes* (24.23%), and *Proteobacteria* (23.31%) comprised the majority of OTUs (88.59%). While at the genus level, *Streptococcus* (28.24%), *Haemophilus* (15.97%), *Prevotella* (14.64%), *Alloprevotella* (5.27%), and *Neisseria* (4.21%) were the most prevalent bacterial taxa throughout the three subjects, which in totality accounted for 69.05% of all salivary bacteria. The relative abundance of these bacterial taxa at the phylum level and genus level are presented in Figure 1. These findings were generally in line with the findings of Belstrøm et al., which indicated the five most predominant genera identified were *Streptococcus*, *Haemophilus*, *Prevotella*, *Rothia*, and *Neisseria*, accounting for around 50% of the identified OTUs [29].

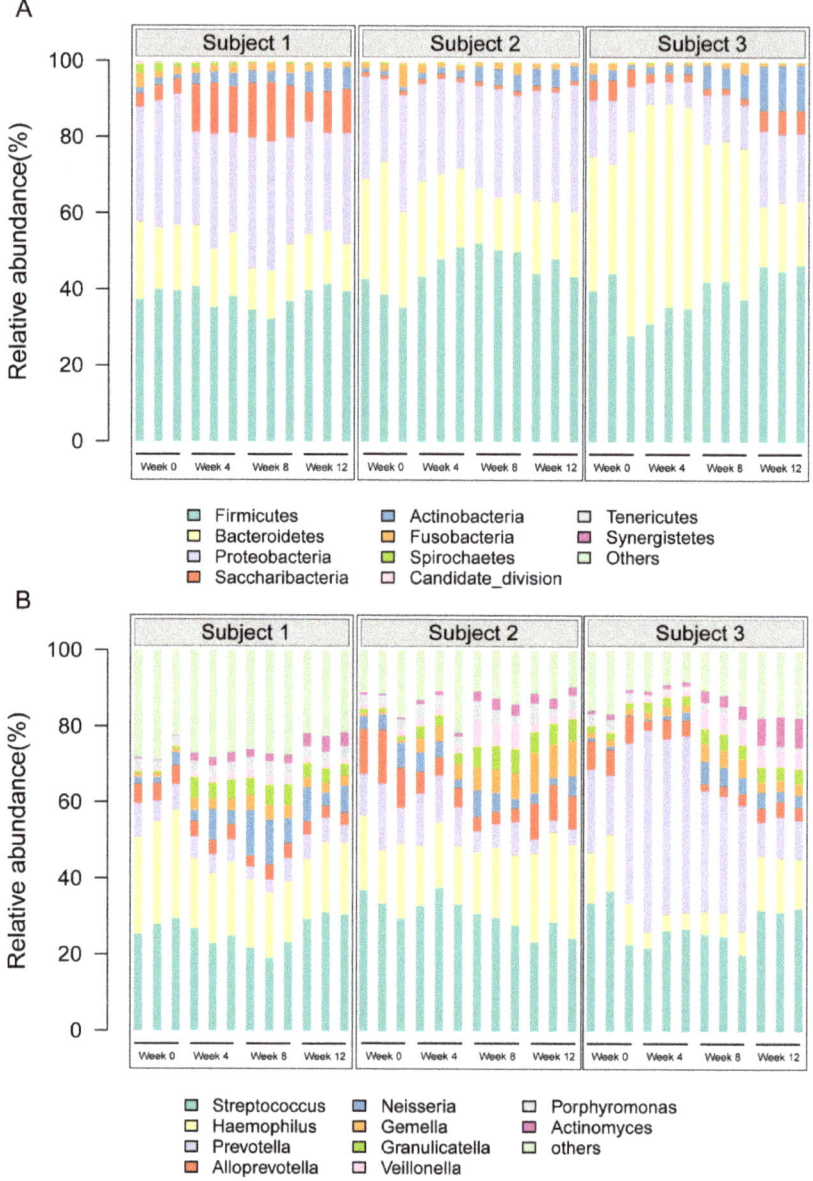

Figure 1. Relative abundances of the most abundant phyla and genera in each salivary sample in the (**A**) phylum level and (**B**) genus level.

3.3. Comparisons of Salivary Bacterial Communities

Based on the relative abundance of all the OTUs, salivary bacterial community diversity (expressed by the Shannon and Simpson indexes) was investigated first, and the results are shown in Table 2. Compared with baseline (week 0), after eight weeks of tea consumption, a remarkable reduction in the community diversity was noticed across the three subjects, with the exception of the Shannon index of subject 3.

Table 2. The temporal changes of the salivary microbial community diversity in each subject.

	Baseline	Tea Intervention		Follow-Up
	Week 0	Week 4	Week 8	Week 12
Subject 1				
Shannon	5.28 ± 0.41 [a]	4.68 ± 0.27 [ab]	4.00 ± 0.39 [b]	4.17 ± 0.40 [b]
Simpson	0.94 ± 0.02 [a]	0.89 ± 0.03 [ab]	0.81 ± 0.04 [b]	0.84 ± 0.06 [b]
Subject 2				
Shannon	4.79 ± 0.58 [a]	4.63 ± 0.22 [ab]	4.02 ± 0.27 [b]	4.37 ± 0.13 [ab]
Simpson	0.91 ± 0.06 [a]	0.88 ± 0.06 [a]	0.83 ± 0.05 [b]	0.90 ± 0.02 [a]
Subject 3				
Shannon	3.99 ± 0.57 [a]	3.93 ± 0.27 [a]	3.90 ± 0.17 [a]	4.07 ± 0.65 [a]
Simpson	0.85 ± 0.10 [a]	0.83 ± 0.03 [a]	0.80 ± 0.03 [b]	0.83 ± 0.09 [a]

Values are expressed as the mean ± SD ($n = 3$). Means with different superscript letters (a, b) within a row suggest significant differences ($p < 0.05$); means with the same superscript letters (a, b) within a row suggest the differences are not significant ($p \geq 0.05$), as determined by Duncan's multiple range test.

In order to adequately compare the homogeneity of salivary bacterial communities among the three subjects, MRPP and Anosim tests were then performed. In the pairwise comparisons, positive delta values from MRPP tests and R values from Anosim tests were observed, which indicated a higher similarity within the groups (Table 3). Thus, diversities of salivary microbiota among individuals were much larger than the variation within individuals over the course of tea consumption.

Table 3. Summary of multiple response permutation procedure (MRPP) and analysis of similarity (Anosim) tests between each subject.

Compared Data Sets	MRPP		Anosim	
	Delta	p-Value	R	p-Value
Subject 1 vs. Subject 2	0.1969	0.001	0.7105	0.001
Subject 1 vs. Subject 3	0.1479	0.001	0.4886	0.001
Subject 2 vs. Subject 3	0.1919	0.001	0.7562	0.001
Subject 1 vs. Subject 2 vs. Subject 3	0.2227	0.001	0.6482	0.001

The general profiles of salivary microbiota of each individual subject at different sampling times were further compared with PCA (Figure 2). For subject 1, the salivary bacterial communities in the baseline period were separated from the tea intervention and follow-up period, while in the follow-up period bacterial communities gathered with those in the tea consumption period. For subject 2, clear distinctions in the bacterial communities were discovered between week 0 and the other experimental periods, while the bacterial communities in week 12 and week 4 were overlapped. In the case of subject 3, relatively higher similarities were found among the different treatment periods, which might suggest a slighter or lower impact of tea consumption on the salivary microbiota.

3.4. Correlation Networks of Salivary Microbiota

Based on the Illumina sequencing results, 67 OTUs were defined as the predominant salivary microbiota of the three subjects, with relative abundance over 0.1%. Pearson's correlations were calculated among the predominant salivary microbiota of each subject, and the strong connections ($|r| > 0.9$ and $p < 0.05$) were further visualized as networks (Figure 3A,C,E). When comparing the networks of the three subjects, subject 1 had the most complicated co-occurrence patterns of salivary bacteria, with a total strong connection number of 128. For subjects 2 and 3, the strong connection numbers were 49 and 41, respectively.

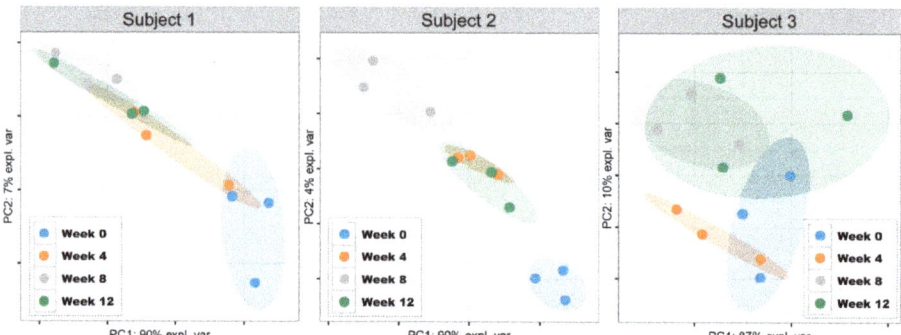

Figure 2. Principal component analysis (PCA) score plots based on the relative abundance of all operational taxonomic units (OTUs) of each subject.

3.5. Hub Salivary Microbiota Identification

The size of each node in the network represents the number of strong connections with other nodes. Thus, the OTUs with a larger node size were identified as the hub salivary microbiota of each subject, which had more connections with other bacteria. In this study, approximately 20 hub OTUs from each subject were intentionally selected. In particular, for subject 1, 21 OTUs were defined as the hub microbiota (Figure 3A). The relative abundance changes of these bacteria were further visualized as a heatmap plot (Figure 3B). Of these, 8 OTUs (OTU 133, 23, 42, 5, 6, 7, 8, and 9) increased after tea intervention, while the remaining 13 OTUs decreased; moreover, OTU 1, 42, and 5 increased during the follow-up period (week 12). For subjects 2 and 3, 20 and 25 OTUs were identified as hub microbiota (Figure 3C,E). The successions of these hub salivary microbiota during the 12-week experimental period are illustrated in Figure 3D,F.

Through a Venn diagram, seven OTUs, including OTU_1 (*Streptococcus* sp.), OTU_133 (*Veillonella* sp.), OTU_23 (*Veillonella* sp.), OTU_33 (*Ruminococcaceae* sp.), OTU_42 (*Actinomyces odontolyticus*), OTU_6 (*Gemella haemolysans*), and OTU_696 (*Haemophilus* sp.), were identified as the shared hub microbiota of the three subjects (Figure 4A). The unique hub salivary microbiome is also shown in Figure 4A. Based on the relative abundance of these shared hub bacteria during the entire experimental period for the three subjects, a PCA plot was further depicted (Figure 4B). A clear separation of the baseline period (week 0) from other score points was observed, which revealed a significant change with regard to these seven OTUs which occurred after tea infusion drinking. The PCA score plots of week 4 and week 8 were gathered into two discrete clusters, which indicated a time-dependent response of these bacteria to tea drinking. For week 12, this cluster was in-between those of week 4 and week 8, indicating a relatively similar bacterial profile pattern in the follow-up period with tea treatment. The temporal shifts of these seven shared hub salivary microbiota during the 12-week experimental period are reflected in Figure 5. In general, compared with the baseline period, in week 4, *Ruminococcaceae* sp. (OTU_33) and *Haemophilus* sp. (OTU_696) were suppressed significantly ($p < 0.05$), while *Veillonella* sp. (OTU_133), *Actinomyces odontolyticus* (OTU_42), and *Gemella haemolysans* (OTU_6) were promoted significantly ($p < 0.05$). After eight weeks of tea consumption, *Streptococcus* sp. (OTU_1), *Ruminococcaceae* sp. (OTU_33), and *Haemophilus* sp. (OTU_696) were suppressed significantly ($p < 0.05$), while *Veillonella* spp. (OTU_133 and OTU_23), *Actinomyces odontolyticus* (OTU_42), and *Gemella haemolysans* (OTU_6) were promoted significantly ($p < 0.05$). In the follow-up period, only *Streptococcus* sp. (OTU_1) was return to its initial level ($p > 0.05$).

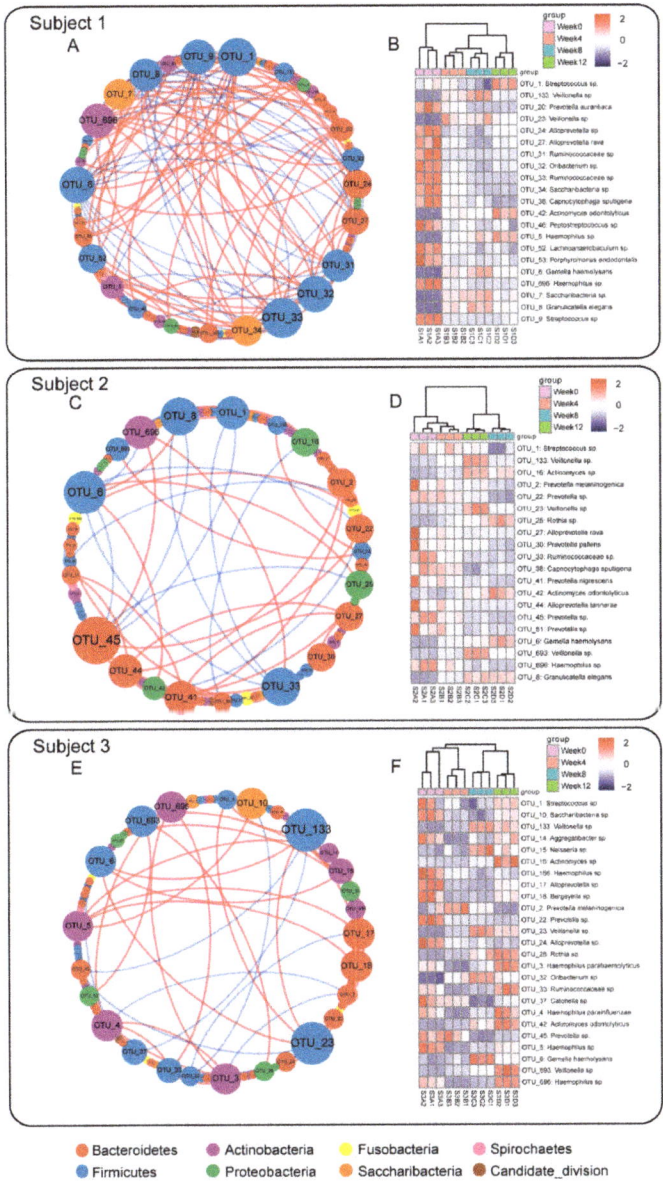

Figure 3. Correlation networks of the predominant salivary microbiota (**A,C,E**) and heatmaps of the hub salivary microbiota (**B,D,F**) in each subject. In correlation networks, each node represents an OTU; the color of nodes indicates the phylum information; the size of nodes represents the number of linkages; lines between nodes represent a strong correlation between these two OTUs ($|r| > 0.9$ and $p < 0.05$, Pearson's correlation); red line represents a positive correlation and blue line represents a negative correlation. The nodes with high strong connection numbers were selected as the "hub microbiota" and their dynamic shifts of relative abundance were further depicted on heatmaps. The color of the data matrix in heatmaps corresponds to the normalized relative abundance of the OTUs; the color bar on the top right indicates the scale.

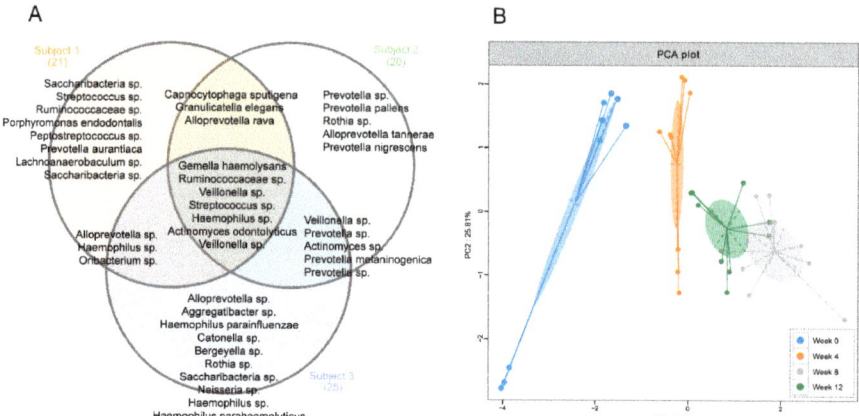

Figure 4. (**A**) The Venn diagram of the hub salivary microbiota in each subject. (**B**) PCA score plots based on the relative abundance of the shared hub microbiota across the three subjects.

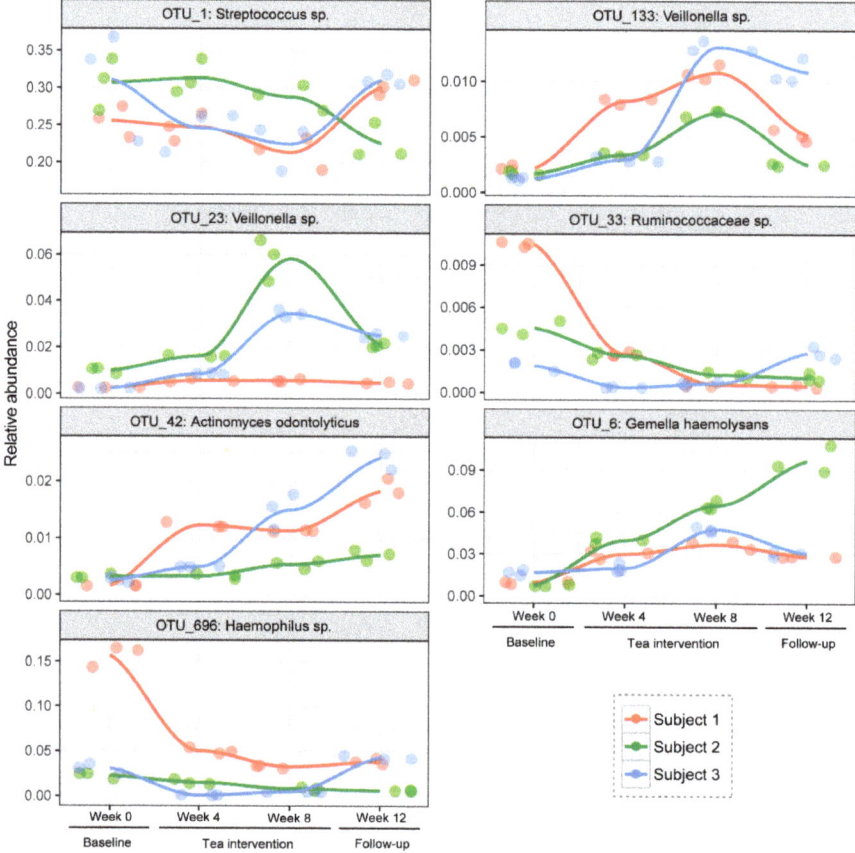

Figure 5. The temporal shifts of the shared hub salivary microbiota during the 12-week experimental period.

4. Discussion

In the present study, an oolong tea infusion containing a total of 2.83 ± 0.02 g/L polyphenols, including catechin, epicatechin, epigallocatechin gallate, and at least 30 other components, was used to evaluate its salivary microbiota modification effect. Three subjects were required to consume 1.0 L of tea infusions daily, which equaled approximately 52 mg/kg body weight of tea polyphenols. The preparation method and intake amount of tea infusions followed the general tea drinking habits of individuals in the southern part of China, which would provide a more pragmatic and appropriate insight. Under this consumption amount, diverse responds of salivary microbiota were observed among the three subjects.

Following the Illumina high-throughput sequencing, a highly diverse salivary bacterial community was observed. A total of 8801 OTUs with a 97% similarity level was identified from the 36 saliva samples and annotated into 25 phyla and 260 genera. In addition to the complexity, a high inter-individual variation in salivary microbiota was also discovered. It was revealed that the salivary microbial communities within the three subjects were significantly distinct from each other, exhibiting host-specific microbiota profiles; their overall collective responses to tea consumption also varied among each participant. The positive delta values from MRPP tests and R values from Anosim tests indicated the differences of salivary microbiota profiles among subjects were far more significant than that among different time points within one subject (Table 3). When all 36 salivary microbiota data sets from the three subjects were depicted into one PCA plot, no clear cluster was observed (Figure S2). The host-specific salivary microbiota were also confirmed by the distinct correlation networks of each participant. These results were consistent with the findings of Belstrøm et al., since the authors confirmed that the five individuals in their study had a personalized salivary bacterial fingerprint [29]. Hall et al. also stated that the oral bacterial community fingerprint varied from person to person in their study [17]. Thus, in order to minimize the inter-individual variations, the data sets from different subjects were analyzed separately, otherwise the effect of tea may be obscured by the inter-individual variations, as shown in Figure S2.

In general, it was revealed that oolong tea consumption led to a profound reduction in diversity of the salivary bacterial communities of subject 1 and subject 2. Takeshita et al. stated in their population-based study that good oral health was associated with a lower phylogenetic diversity of the salivary microbiome [5]. Moreover, Vestman et al. reported that the diversity of the tooth biofilm samples was reduced after probiotics supplementation [30]. The increase of diversity of gut microbiota is normally associated with better gut health conditions, such as through the extension of the functional genes for facilitation of the absorption of nutrients and energy, or for appropriate development of immunity. In contrast to the commensal microbiota residents in the intestinal tract, which typically live in harmony with the host, the oral microbiota is responsible for the two most common diseases, including dental caries and periodontal diseases [31]. The increase of diversity in salivary microbiota may be associated with the flourish of dental plaque which resulted from the accumulation of attached bacteria, and thus increase the risk of dental caries and periodontal diseases; while, the decrease in taxonomic diversity in saliva may indicate the shrinking of bacterial communities in dental plaque biofilms, and thus lead to healthier oral ecological conditions. However, for subject 3, the decrease of the salivary microbial community diversity was not significant, except for Simpson index of week 8, which might indicate a lower modulation effect of tea on subject 3. Furthermore, according to PCA, significant overall shifts of salivary microbiota composition were noted in subjects 1 and 2. However, in the case of subject 3, a higher variation was discovered amongst different sampling time points, which may also suggest a lower effectiveness of tea consumption upon the salivary microbiota of subject 3.

The oral cavity, as the portal of entry to the gastrointestinal tract, is one of the most complex microbial colony sites within the human body [32]. In order to better understand the complex ecologic system, a correlation network was employed in this study to simplify and visualize the co-occurrence patterns of salivary bacteria. The bacteria taxa with robust connections with other salivary bacteria were defined as "hub salivary bacteria". Subsequently, via a heatmap plot, the temporal dynamic of each individual hub salivary bacteria was clearly presented. Afterwards, through a Venn diagram, the shared hub microbiota across the three subjects were further identified. Separated correlation network analysis revealed the detailed influence of tea consumption on the salivary microbiota composition within the same contactable environment. Thus, it minimized the inter-individual variations between subjects. While, an additional Venn diagram further helped in seeking the common influences of tea consumption.

In particular, seven shared hub OTUs across the three subjects were identified from the highly complex and personalized oral ecosystem. Notably, OTU_1 (*Streptococcus* sp.), as the most predominant taxon, also acted as a shared hub microbiota and favorably interacted with other oral bacteria. Due to the biofilm formation and acid production ability of *Streptococcus*, multiple members of this genus, including *Streptococcus mutans*, *Streptococcus sobrinus*, *Streptococcus salivarius*, *Streptococcus constellatus*, and *Streptococcus parasanguinis*, were considered as opportunistic pathogens [33]. With regard to the shifts of *Streptococcus* sp., a significant decrease (-16.94%, $p = 0.035$) was found after eight weeks of tea consumption. Therefore, a *Streptococcus* inhibitory effect of tea was observed in this study, and the effect may assist in the prevention of dental caries. There is a preponderance of evidence to support the beneficial role of tea in protecting against this oral pathogen. Narotzki et al. reviewed the clinical and biological studies regarding the correlation between green tea and oral health and concluded that green tea may reduce dental caries through bacterial growth repression and enzyme activity inhibition [14]. With the exception of green tea, it has also been reported that black tea extracts could inhibit *S. mutans* adhesion in vitro [34]. Kawarai et al. compared the *S. mutans* biofilm formation inhibitory effect of Assam tea (a black tea variety) and green tea and ascertained that Assam tea exhibited a stronger biofilm inhibition activity than green tea [35]. The inhibitory activity of specific teas against oral pathogens are commonly attributed to the phenolic components within the tea [14].

Similar inhibitory effects were also observed on OTU_33 (*Ruminococcaceae* sp.) and OTU_696 (*Haemophilus* sp.), both of which were also hub microbiota across the three subjects. *Haemophilus* are a common bacteria which inhabit the mouth, vagina, and intestinal tract. The genus includes commensal organisms, along with some pathogenic species such as *H. influenzae* and *H. ducreyi*. The inhibitory effect of tea on *Haemophilus* may also reduce the risk of infection. *Ruminococcaceae*, one of the most typical gut microbiotas, can be found in significant numbers in the intestines of humans. However, the biological meaning regarding the depletion of this bacterium induced by tea drinking was not clear.

Along with oolong tea consumption, a significant elevation of OTU_133 (*Veillonella* sp.), OTU_23 (*Veillonella* sp.), OTU_42 (*Actinomyces odontolyticus*), and OTU_6 (*Gemella haemolysans*), which were all demonstrated as robust network nodes across the three subjects, was observed in this study. Lim et al. illustrated a significant negative association between *Haemophilus* and *Veillonella* [36], which was consistent with our findings. Furthermore, it was reported that the establishment of some certain oral commensals was linked to oral health, such as the bacterial species belonging to *Neisseria*, *Veillonella*, and *Actinomyces* [37], although details regarding the exact mechanisms are not yet available. Moreover, the elevated effect on these four hub bacteria continued throughout the follow-up period, which demonstrated the sustained effect of tea drinking.

With regard to the mechanisms behind the modification effect of tea on salivary microbiota, several hypotheses have been invoked to account for this particular effect: (i) tea polyphenols possess antimicrobial properties, which are believed to aid in the inhibition of certain bacteria, including some pathogens [13,14]; (ii) tea polyphenols as antioxidants may alleviate oral oxidative stress and inflammation, which may further impact the oral immune system and induce a drift of the bacterial community [14]; (iii) tea polyphenols can precipitate salivary proteins and inhibit the activity of salivary alpha-amylase, and thus, induce the decrease of fermentation of carbohydrates involved in caries formation [38]. However, the precise mechanism is still ambiguous, resulting in the necessity for further studies. Numerous epidemiologic studies and clinical trials have validated that regular tea consumption could reduce the risk of cardiovascular disease, including coronary heart disease, stroke, and peripheral arterial disease [39]. Recent studies show a correlation between periodontal disease and cardiovascular disease [40,41]. Thus, from the perspective of alleviating systematic inflammatory and immunological processes, explicating the underlying mechanisms (e.g., to link the levels of endogenous mediators, such as endothelin [42] and vitamins [9] of tea consumption may open an innovative avenue toward the development of new antibiotics with good safety and tolerability margin.

It was also acknowledged that the inadequate number of subjects in this study might limit the statistical analysis. As explained previously, using limited subjects and following the time course of each individual may help to minimize the inter-individual variations. However, further studies with larger sample sizes are warranted to validate these findings.

5. Conclusions

In summary, using three healthy adult volunteers as our subjects, our study demonstrated that a daily consumption of 1.0 L oolong tea for eight weeks caused a reduction in bacterial community diversity, as well as the disturbance of hub salivary bacterium with strong connections to other salivary microbiota. Additionally, it was also noticed that large inter-individual variations were found, implying diverse responses to oolong tea consumption may exist among subjects. Larger sample sizes and more in-depth mechanism studies are necessary to further clarify and elucidate the physiological relevance of the shifts of salivary microbiota to the oral health of the host.

Supplementary Materials: The following are available online at http://www.mdpi.com/2072-6643/12/4/966/s1, Figure S1: Chromatograms obtained from oolong tea infusion, using UHPLC Q-TOF-MS/MS in negative and positive ion modes, Figure S2: PCA score plot based on the relative abundance of all OTUs of the three subjects, Table S1: Summary of the sequencing results of all salivary samples.

Author Contributions: Conceptualization, Z.L., W.Z., and L.N.; formal analysis, Z.L. and H.G.; main funding acquisition, L.N.; investigation, Z.L., H.G., and W.Z.; project administration, L.N.; supervision, L.N.; visualization, Z.L.; writing—original draft, Z.L.; writing—review and editing, Z.L., W.Z., and L.N. All authors read and approved the final manuscript.

Funding: This study was supported by the National Key Research and Development Plan of China (no. 2016YFD0400801).

Acknowledgments: The authors thank Jun Lin, Fujian Agriculture and Forestry University, for his excellent technical assistance.

Conflicts of Interest: The authors declare no conflicts of interest.

References

1. Jenkinson, H.F.; Lamont, R.J. Oral microbial communities in sickness and in health. *Trends Microbiol.* **2005**, *13*, 589–595. [CrossRef]
2. Velden, U.V.D.; Winkelhoff, A.J.V.; Abbas, F.; Graaff, J.D. The habitat of periodontopathic micro-organisms. *J. Clin. Periodontol.* **1986**, *13*, 243–248. [CrossRef]
3. Yang, F.; Zeng, X.; Ning, K.; Liu, K.-L.; Lo, C.-C.; Wang, W.; Chen, J.; Wang, D.; Huang, R.; Chang, X. Saliva microbiomes distinguish caries-active from healthy human populations. *ISME J.* **2012**, *6*, 1–10. [CrossRef] [PubMed]
4. Lazarevic, V.; Whiteson, K.; Hernandez, D.; François, P.; Schrenzel, J. Study of inter-and intra-individual variations in the salivary microbiota. *BMC Genom.* **2010**, *11*, 523. [CrossRef] [PubMed]
5. Takeshita, T.; Kageyama, S.; Furuta, M.; Tsuboi, H.; Takeuchi, K.; Shibata, Y.; Shimazaki, Y.; Akifusa, S.; Ninomiya, T.; Kiyohara, Y. Bacterial diversity in saliva and oral health-related conditions: The Hisayama Study. *Sci. Rep.* **2016**, *6*, 22164. [CrossRef] [PubMed]
6. Chinsembu, K.C. Plants and other natural products used in the management of oral infections and improvement of oral health. *Acta Trop.* **2016**, *154*, 6–18. [CrossRef] [PubMed]
7. Musarra-Pizzo, M.; Ginestra, G.; Smeriglio, A.; Pennisi, R.; Sciortino, M.T.; Mandalari, G. The antimicrobial and antiviral activity of polyphenols from almond (Prunus dulcis L.) skin. *Nutrients* **2019**, *11*, 2355. [CrossRef] [PubMed]
8. Tsou, S.-H.; Hu, S.-W.; Yang, J.-J.; Yan, M.; Lin, Y.-Y. Potential Oral Health Care Agent from Coffee against Virulence Factor of Periodontitis. *Nutrients* **2019**, *11*, 2235. [CrossRef]

9. Isola, G.; Polizzi, A.; Muraglie, S.; Leonardi, R.; Lo Giudice, A. Assessment of Vitamin C and Antioxidant Profiles in Saliva and Serum in Patients with Periodontitis and Ischemic Heart Disease. *Nutrients* **2019**, *11*, 2956. [CrossRef]
10. Isola, G. Current Evidence of Natural Agents in Oral and Periodontal Health. *Nutrients* **2020**, *12*, 585. [CrossRef]
11. Chun, O.K.; Chung, S.J.; Song, W.O. Estimated dietary flavonoid intake and major food sources of US adults. *J. Nutr.* **2007**, *137*, 1244–1252. [CrossRef] [PubMed]
12. Ferrazzano, G.F.; Roberto, L.; Amato, I.; Cantile, T.; Sangianantoni, G.; Ingenito, A. Antimicrobial properties of green tea extract against cariogenic microflora: An in vivo study. *J. Med. Food* **2011**, *14*, 907–911. [CrossRef] [PubMed]
13. Ferrazzano, G.F.; Amato, I.; Ingenito, A.; De Natale, A.; Pollio, A. Anti-cariogenic effects of polyphenols from plant stimulant beverages (cocoa, coffee, tea). *Fitoterapia* **2009**, *80*, 255–262. [CrossRef] [PubMed]
14. Narotzki, B.; Reznick, A.Z.; Aizenbud, D.; Levy, Y. Green tea: A promising natural product in oral health. *Arch. Oral Biol.* **2012**, *57*, 429–435. [CrossRef] [PubMed]
15. Liu, Z.; Chen, Z.; Guo, H.; He, D.; Zhao, H.; Wang, Z.; Zhang, W.; Liao, L.; Zhang, C.; Ni, L. The modulatory effect of infusions of green tea, oolong tea, and black tea on gut microbiota in high-fat-induced obese mice. *Food Funct.* **2016**, *7*, 4869–4879. [CrossRef]
16. Liu, Z.; Bruins, M.E.; Ni, L.; Vincken, J.-P. Green and black tea phenolics: Bioavailability, transformation by colonic microbiota, and modulation of colonic microbiota. *J. Agric. Food Chem.* **2018**, *66*, 8469–8477. [CrossRef]
17. Hall, M.W.; Singh, N.; Ng, K.F.; Lam, D.K.; Goldberg, M.B.; Tenenbaum, H.C.; Neufeld, J.D.; Beiko, R.; Senadheera, D.B. Inter-personal diversity and temporal dynamics of dental, tongue, and salivary microbiota in the healthy oral cavity. *NPJ Biofilm. Microbiomes* **2017**, *3*, 2. [CrossRef]
18. Obanda, M.; Owuor, P.O.; Taylor, S.J. Flavanol composition and caffeine content of green leaf as quality potential indicators of Kenyan black teas. *J. Sci. Food Agric.* **1997**, *74*, 209–215. [CrossRef]
19. Magoč, T.; Salzberg, S.L. FLASH: Fast length adjustment of short reads to improve genome assemblies. *Bioinformatics* **2011**, *27*, 2957–2963. [CrossRef]
20. Caporaso, J.G.; Kuczynski, J.; Stombaugh, J.; Bittinger, K.; Bushman, F.D.; Costello, E.K.; Fierer, N.; Pena, A.G.; Goodrich, J.K.; Gordon, J.I. QIIME allows analysis of high-throughput community sequencing data. *Nat. Methods* **2010**, *7*, 335. [CrossRef]
21. Bokulich, N.A.; Subramanian, S.; Faith, J.J.; Gevers, D.; Gordon, J.I.; Knight, R.; Mills, D.A.; Caporaso, J.G. Quality-filtering vastly improves diversity estimates from Illumina amplicon sequencing. *Nat. Methods* **2013**, *10*, 57. [CrossRef] [PubMed]
22. Edgar, R.C. UPARSE: Highly accurate OTU sequences from microbial amplicon reads. *Nat. Methods* **2013**, *10*, 996. [CrossRef] [PubMed]
23. DeSantis, T.Z.; Hugenholtz, P.; Larsen, N.; Rojas, M.; Brodie, E.L.; Keller, K.; Huber, T.; Dalevi, D.; Hu, P.; Andersen, G.L. Greengenes, a chimera-checked 16S rRNA gene database and workbench compatible with ARB. *Appl. Environ. Microbiol.* **2006**, *72*, 5069–5072. [CrossRef] [PubMed]
24. Chen, T.; Yu, W.-H.; Izard, J.; Baranova, O.V.; Lakshmanan, A.; Dewhirst, F.E. The Human Oral Microbiome Database: A web accessible resource for investigating oral microbe taxonomic and genomic information. *Database* **2010**, *2010*. [CrossRef] [PubMed]
25. Bastian, M.; Heymann, S.; Jacomy, M. Gephi: An open source software for exploring and manipulating networks. *ICWSM* **2009**, *8*, 361–362.
26. Faust, K.; Lima-Mendez, G.; Lerat, J.-S.; Sathirapongsasuti, J.F.; Knight, R.; Huttenhower, C.; Lenaerts, T.; Raes, J. Cross-biome comparison of microbial association networks. *Front. Microbiol.* **2015**, *6*, 1200. [CrossRef]
27. Layeghifard, M.; Hwang, D.M.; Guttman, D.S. Disentangling interactions in the microbiome: A network perspective. *Trends Microbiol.* **2017**, *25*, 217–228. [CrossRef]
28. Heberle, H.; Meirelles, G.V.; da Silva, F.R.; Telles, G.P.; Minghim, R. InteractiVenn: A web-based tool for the analysis of sets through Venn diagrams. *BMC Bioinform.* **2015**, *16*, 169. [CrossRef]
29. Belstrøm, D.; Holmstrup, P.; Bardow, A.; Kokaras, A.; Fiehn, N.-E.; Paster, B.J. Temporal stability of the salivary microbiota in oral health. *PLoS ONE* **2016**, *11*, e0147472. [CrossRef]

30. Romani Vestman, N.; Chen, T.; Lif Holgerson, P.; Öhman, C.; Johansson, I. Oral microbiota shift after 12-week supplementation with Lactobacillus reuteri DSM 17938 and PTA 5289; a randomized control trial. *PLoS ONE* **2015**, *10*, e0125812. [CrossRef]
31. Wade, W.G. The oral microbiome in health and disease. *Pharmacol. Res.* **2013**, *69*, 137–143. [CrossRef] [PubMed]
32. Consortium, H.M.P. Structure, function and diversity of the healthy human microbiome. *Nature* **2012**, *486*, 207–214.
33. Jiang, W.; Ling, Z.; Lin, X.; Chen, Y.; Zhang, J.; Yu, J.; Xiang, C.; Chen, H. Pyrosequencing analysis of oral microbiota shifting in various caries states in childhood. *Microb. Ecol.* **2014**, *67*, 962–969. [CrossRef] [PubMed]
34. Limsong, J.; Benjavongkulchai, E.; Kuvatanasuchati, J. Inhibitory effect of some herbal extracts on adherence of Streptococcus mutans. *J. Ethnopharmacol.* **2004**, *92*, 281–289. [CrossRef]
35. Kawarai, T.; Narisawa, N.; Yoneda, S.; Tsutsumi, Y.; Ishikawa, J.; Hoshino, Y.; Senpuku, H. Inhibition of Streptococcus mutans biofilm formation using extracts from Assam tea compared to green tea. *Arch. Oral Biol.* **2016**, *68*, 73–82. [CrossRef]
36. Lim, M.Y.; Yoon, H.S.; Rho, M.; Sung, J.; Song, Y.-M.; Lee, K.; Ko, G. Analysis of the association between host genetics, smoking, and sputum microbiota in healthy humans. *Sci. Rep.* **2016**, *6*, 23745. [CrossRef]
37. Paropkari, A.D.; Leblebicioglu, B.; Christian, L.M.; Kumar, P.S. Smoking, pregnancy and the subgingival microbiome. *Sci. Rep.* **2016**, *6*, 30388. [CrossRef]
38. Hara, K.; Ohara, M.; Hayashi, I.; Hino, T.; Nishimura, R.; Iwasaki, Y.; Ogawa, T.; Ohyama, Y.; Sugiyama, M.; Amano, H. The green tea polyphenol (−)-epigallocatechin gallate precipitates salivary proteins including alpha-amylase: Biochemical implications for oral health. *Eur. J. Oral Sci.* **2012**, *120*, 132–139. [CrossRef]
39. Khan, N.; Mukhtar, H. Tea polyphenols in promotion of human health. *Nutrients* **2019**, *11*, 39. [CrossRef]
40. Isola, G.; Alibrandi, A.; Currò, M.; Matarese, M.; Ricca, S.; Matarese, G.; Ientile, R.; Kocher, T. Evaluation of salivary and serum ADMA levels in patients with periodontal and cardiovascular disease as subclinical marker of cardiovascular risk. *J. Periodontol.* **2019**. [CrossRef]
41. Isola, G.; Giudice, A.L.; Polizzi, A.; Alibrandi, A.; Patini, R.; Ferlito, S. Periodontitis and Tooth Loss Have Negative Systemic Impact on Circulating Progenitor Cell Levels: A Clinical Study. *Genes* **2019**, *10*, 1022. [CrossRef] [PubMed]
42. Isola, G.; Polizzi, A.; Alibrandi, A.; Indelicato, F.; Ferlito, S. Analysis of Endothelin-1 concentrations in individuals with periodontitis. *Sci. Rep.* **2020**, *10*, 1652. [CrossRef] [PubMed]

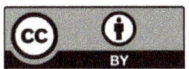

© 2020 by the authors. Licensee MDPI, Basel, Switzerland. This article is an open access article distributed under the terms and conditions of the Creative Commons Attribution (CC BY) license (http://creativecommons.org/licenses/by/4.0/).

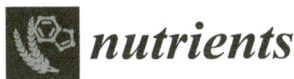

Article

Assessment of vitamin C and Antioxidant Profiles in Saliva and Serum in Patients with Periodontitis and Ischemic Heart Disease

Gaetano Isola [1,*], Alessandro Polizzi [1], Simone Muraglie [1], Rosalia Leonardi [1] and Antonino Lo Giudice [1,2]

[1] Department of General Surgery and Surgical-Medical Specialties, School of Dentistry, University of Catania, Via S. Sofia 78, 95124 Catania, Italy; alexpoli345@gmail.com (A.P.); simonemuraglie@live.it (S.M.); rleonard@unict.it (R.L.); nino.logiudice@gmail.com (A.L.G.)
[2] Department of Biomedical and Dental Sciences and Morphofunctional Imaging, School of Dentistry, University of Messina, 98125 Messina, Italy
* Correspondence: gaetano.isola@unict.it; Tel./Fax: +39-0957435359

Received: 8 November 2019; Accepted: 29 November 2019; Published: 4 December 2019

Abstract: vitamin C and antioxidants play a crucial role in endothelial function and may be a link for the known interaction of periodontitis and ischemic heart disease (CAD). This pilot study evaluates the association of gingival health, periodontitis, CAD, or both conditions with salivary and serum vitamin C and antioxidant levels. The clinical and periodontal characteristics, serum, and saliva samples were collected from 36 patients with periodontitis, 35 patients with CAD, 36 patients with periodontitis plus CAD, and 36 healthy controls. Levels of vitamin C, antioxidants, and C-reactive protein (hs-CRP) were assessed with a commercially available kit. The median concentrations of salivary and serum vitamin C and antioxidants (α-tocopherol, β-carotene, lutein, and lycopene) were significantly lower in the CAD group ($p < 0.001$) and in the periodontitis plus CAD group ($p < 0.001$) compared to periodontitis patients and controls. In univariate models, periodontitis ($p = 0.034$), CAD ($p < 0.001$), and hs-CRP ($p < 0.001$) were significantly negatively associated with serum vitamin C; whereas, in a multivariate model, only hs-CRP remained a significant predictor of serum vitamin C ($p < 0.001$). In a multivariate model, the significant predictors of salivary vitamin C levels were triglycerides ($p = 0.028$) and hs-CRP ($p < 0.001$). Patients with CAD and periodontitis plus CAD presented lower levels of salivary and serum vitamin C compared to healthy subjects and periodontitis patients. hs-CRP was a significant predictor of decreased salivary and serum vitamin C levels.

Keywords: vitamin C; retinol; α-carotene; β-carotene; β-cryptoxanthin; γ-tocopherol; lutein; zeaxanthin; lycopene; periodontitis; ischemic heart disease; C-reactive protein; cardiovascular disease; clinical trial

1. Introduction

About 50% of adults in the United States of America (USA), aged over 30 years, are affected by periodontitis, and almost 10% of the world population have a severe form of periodontal disease [1,2]. Periodontitis can be defined as a chronic inflammatory multifactorial disease caused by periodontal bacteria that determine the destruction of the tooth-supporting tissues, including alveolar bone, and which can lead to tooth loss [3]. Some observational studies during the last few decades have shown a direct and positive association between periodontitis and coronary heart disease, known also as ischemic heart disease (CAD), including myocardial infarction, stroke, and cardiovascular disease (CVD) [4,5]. More specifically, recent large cohort studies and a systematic review highlighted a positive graded association between periodontitis and increased risk of stroke and CAD [6–8].

The etiology of periodontitis comprises inflammatory and immunological processes that cause dysregulation in the host response due to the superinfection of periodontal bacteria [9]. Moreover, periodontitis has been positively associated with higher serum levels of different inflammatory biomarkers, such as interleukin 6 (IL-6), IL-17, C-reactive protein, and prostaglandins [10].

vitamin C has been shown, together with some other antioxidant agents, to be an endogenous modulator of the metabolism of nitric oxide (NO) and subsequent endothelium-dependent vasodilation [11]. NO is one of the important mediators that regulate function and vasodilatation of the endothelium, because it controls the level of inflammation in the vessels, vascular tone, and cell proliferation, and it modulates the release of different growth factors [12]. vitamin C has been extensively used to evaluate and predict early signs of endothelial dysfunction and CAD events [13]. A prospective study on 200 patients with heart failure showed that patients with high serum vitamin C deficiency moderated the relationship between inflammation and CAD events [14]. Furthermore, a multi-trial study on 134 subjects with CAD showed a therapeutic use of vitamins C and E against the reperfusion damage produced during angioplasty [15].

Few reports have associated periodontitis with CAD, endothelial dysfunction, and augmented the risk of CVD [16–18]. It has previously been hypothesized that several inflammatory mediators are systemically released during periodontitis, including CRP, metalloproteases, and prostaglandins, into the bloodstream and decrease the production of NO [19]. The reduced production of NO negatively impacts the vascular endothelial cells, whose impairment determines, finally, endothelial dysfunction, vasodilatation, and CAD [20,21]. Hence, this has aroused interest in assessing possible oral factors that influence and regulate endothelial changes as subclinical signs of CAD.

Previous studies have demonstrated an indirect association between high serum vitamin C and a direct association between high CRP levels and consequent endothelial damage in patients with periodontitis [22,23].

The local production of NO has an essential role in the development and progression of periodontitis. Both increases and decreases in the production of salivary NO metabolites during periodontitis in gingival tissue against periodontal bacteria and periodontal tissues have been reported to be associated with impaired endothelium-dependent vasodilatation [24]. More specifically, it has been shown that vitamin C and several antioxidants act as a competitive stimulator of the NO synthase, and that lower serum vitamin C levels have been reported in several metabolic disorders, including periodontitis [25,26].

All of these studies were performed only on serum vitamin C. To date, few studies have evaluated salivary vitamin C levels during periodontitis. Moreover, there are insufficient data on the association of periodontitis on both serum and salivary vitamin C levels during periodontitis and CAD.

The aims of this study were to evaluate a possible association of gingival health, periodontitis, CAD, or a combination of both diseases on saliva and serum vitamin C and antioxidant levels. Moreover, the association between both saliva and serum vitamin C levels were assessed, and whether salivary or serum vitamin C levels were mediated by serum CRP in patients with periodontitis and with CAD.

2. Materials and Methods

2.1. Study Design

The study population consisted of 309 patients with periodontitis, CAD, and healthy controls selected among those who attended the Department of Periodontology, School of Dentistry, from June 2016 to October 2018. Groups were selected from a prespecified age range (40–60) and sex so that a similar proportion to the cases fall into the categories defined by the selection variable (sex and age in this study). Fifty percent of the cases and controls were males aged 45–58 years.

The study was performed by the Declaration of Helsinki, revised in 2016 by medical research. Ethical approval was obtained from the local IRB of the University of Messina (012-2016). The study was registered at clinicaltrials.gov (NCT03873789). Written informed consent was obtained from each patient about the study characteristics and possible risks of the study. This study followed the STROBE guidelines for the strengthening of reporting of observational studies (Table S1) [27].

Inclusion criteria for the periodontitis group were: (1) Presence of at least 16 teeth; (2) a minimum of 40% of sites with clinical attachment level (CAL) ≥2 mm and probing depth (PD) ≥4 mm [28]; (3) presence of at least one site for each quadrant with ≥2 mm of crestal alveolar bone loss verified on digital periapical radiographs; and (4) presence of ≥40% sites with bleeding on probing (BOP) [29]. Healthy individuals presented no systemic disease, ≤10% sites with BOP, no sites with PD ≥4 mm or CAL ≥4 mm, no sites with BOP [29] or radiographic signs of bone loss.

Inclusion criteria for the CAD group were: At least ≥18 years old with a diagnosis of CVD, ≥50% of stenosis of at least one coronary artery verified by coronary angiography or a coronary artery bypass surgery, or past or current percutaneous coronary intervention [30]. Moreover, information on previous medical conditions, cardiovascular risk factors, medications, electrocardiography, echocardiography, and coronary angiogram results were collected. The inclusion criteria for the periodontitis + CAD group were based on the same criteria of the single periodontitis and CAD groups but combined.

The exclusion criteria for all patients were: (1) Use of contraceptives; (2) use of antibiotics, immunosuppressive or anti-inflammatory drugs throughout the last three months prior to the study; (3) status of pregnancy or lactation; (4) previous history of excessive drinking; (5) allergy to local anaesthetic; (6) use of drugs that may potentially determine gingival hyperplasia such as Hydantoin, Nifedipine, Cyclosporin A, or similar drugs; (7) periodontal therapy throughout the last three months prior to the study.

After a first screening, 166 patients were excluded from the final sample because they did not meet the inclusion criteria (n = 141), declined to participate (n = 14), or did not attend the first appointment (n = 11). Finally, for this study, 36 patients with periodontitis, 35 patients with CAD, 36 patients with periodontitis plus CAD, and 36 healthy subjects were finally enrolled (Figure 1).

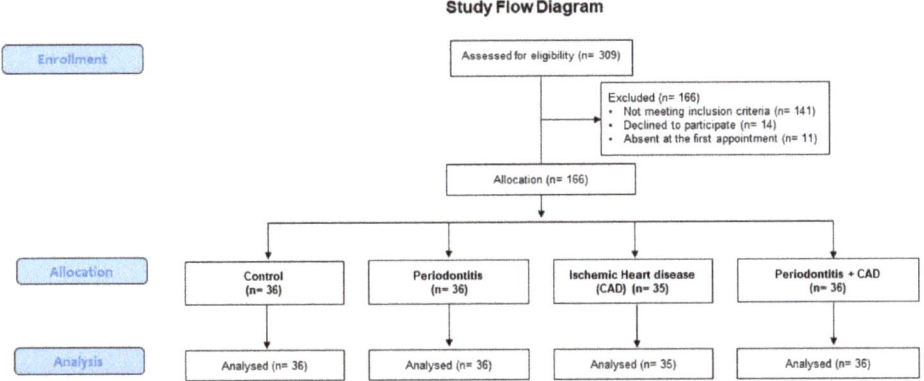

Figure 1. Flowchart of the study.

The demographic (level of education), clinical and medical characteristics (sex, age, body mass index, hypertension, diabetes, dyslipidemia, previous CVD events), and medications were assessed in all enrolled subjects. The presence of diabetes mellitus was based on the history of the patient or a fasting blood glucose ≥126 mg/dL. Body Mass Index (BMI) was estimated on the weight of the patient divided by the square of the patient's height, i.e., kilogram per square meter (kg/m^2).

The periodontal evaluation comprised probing depth (PD), clinical attachment loss (CAL), bleeding on probing (BOP), and plaque score (PI) [31], and the presence of bleeding was recorded up to 30 s after probing. CAL was recorded as PD plus recession, with the cementoenamel junction as a reference for CAL measurements. All clinical periodontal parameters were recorded, in all patients, at six sites per tooth on all teeth present, excluding third molars, by two independent calibrated examiners (a principal examiner and a second control examiner) not involved in the subsequent data analysis with a manual periodontal probe (UNC-15, Hu-Friedy, Chicago, IL, USA). The inter- and intra-examiner reliability of the outcomes PD and CAL were assessed using the intraclass correlation coefficient (ICC). The inter-examiner reliability resulted in an agreement for PD (ICC = 0.817) and CAL (ICC = 0.826), denoting a reasonable degree of reliability for both parameters. The intra-examiner reliability of PD and CAL was performed only on 20 selected patients (five patients per group chosen randomly) for both examiners. The intra-examiner reliability for the first examiner resulted in an agreement for PD (ICC = 0.834) and CAL (ICC = 0.809), and for the second examiner, it resulted in an agreement for PD (ICC = 0.851) and CAL (ICC = 0.819), denoting a reasonable degree of reliability for both parameters.

A power analysis was performed to calculate the minimum sample size required. The sample size was established considering a number of groups equal to 4, an effect size of 0.30 for vitamin C (that represented the primary outcome variable), an expected standard deviation of 1.5 [25], a 2-sided significance level of 0.05, and a power of 80%. It was determined that approximately 32 patients per group would be needed. Thus, it was estimated that 128 subjects were needed to ensure a power level of 80%. One hundred and forty-three patients were enrolled so that the study achieved a power of 83%. Power and sample size calculations were performed using statistical software (G*Power version 3.1.9.4, Universitat Dusseldorf, Germany).

2.2. vitamin C Assessment in Saliva and Serum

Fasting samples were collected in all subjects between 8:00 and 10:00 am. Participants were asked to refrain from eating, drinking, chewing gum, brushing teeth, as well from using any mouthwashes, in the last 12 h before the sampling.

The venous puncture was performed, and blood samples were collected, cooled on ice immediately, and centrifuged at 4 °C (800× g per 10 min). Serum samples were stabilized immediately using metaphosphoric acid in order to avoid oxidization of vitamin C. To collect saliva, subjects were asked to chew on a cotton roll for 2 min, and saliva samples were collected using Salivette collection devices (Sarsted, Verona, Italy) and immediately centrifuged at 4 °C (1000× g per 2 min). Serum and saliva samples were stored at −20 °C until analysis.

Levels of vitamin C and antioxidants (retinol, α-carotene, β-carotene, γ-tocopherol, β-cryptoxanthin, lutein, zeaxanthin, and lycopene) were assessed by use of the commercially available kit for high-performance liquid chromatography (HPLC) measurements (Eureka, Ancona, Italy). In fasting conditions, levels of C-reactive protein (hs-CRP) were assessed by a commercially available nephelometric assay. An hs-CRP level higher than 3 mg/L was associated with an increased risk of CAD. Plasma lipids and glucose were determined by routine methods.

2.3. Statistical Analysis

The numerical data are expressed as median, 25% and 75% percentiles, and categorical variables as number and percentage. The Kruskal–Wallis test was applied in order to compare the four groups with regard to all numerical variables, and the Mann–Whitney test in order to perform two-by-two comparisons between groups. Since most of the examined variables (e.g., triglycerides, fasting glucose, and all periodontal variables) did not present normal distribution, as verified by a Kolmogorov–Smirnov test, the analysis was performed by non-parametric tests. For these multiple comparisons, Bonferroni's correction was applied, for which the significant alpha level 0.050 was divided by the number of possible comparisons ($n = 6$), so the "adjusted" significance level for this analysis was equal to $0.050/6 = 0.008$. A p-trend was performed with the Jonckheere–Terpstra Test for serum and salivary vitamin C levels to assess whether the vitamin C levels were significantly increased in healthy, periodontitis, CAD, and periodontitis + CAD patients. The Spearman correlation test was applied to determine the existence of any significant interdependence between hs-CRP, serum, and salivary vitamin C.

In all enrolled subjects, univariate and multivariable linear regression models were performed in order to assess the dependence of salivary and serum vitamin C levels on potentially explicative variables such as age, gender, education, socioeconomic status (SES), BMI, CRP, triglycerides, total cholesterol, and antioxidants. In the final multivariate model, only age, gender, education, and SES were included as confounders, and tests were carried out to analyze if periodontitis, CAD, and hs-CRP influenced serum vitamin C levels. The same analysis was performed for salivary vitamin C as an outcome. Statistical analyses were performed using statistical software (SPSS 22.0 for Windows package (SPS Srl, Bologna, Italy)). A p-value < 0.05 was considered statistically significant.

3. Results

The patient characteristics and biochemical parameters of the recruited subjects are summarized in Table 1. Controls and patients were matched for age and gender, and there were no significant differences between the distribution of education levels or median values (25% and 75% percentiles) of BMI, triglycerides, or total cholesterol between the groups (Table 1). Increased values of hs-CRP were observed among patients with periodontitis, CAD, and periodontitis + CAD in comparison with healthy subjects ($p < 0.001$). Patients with CAD and periodontitis + CAD had a similar proportion of previous CVD events (atrial fibrillation, angina pectoris, stroke, heart failure) and took more CVD drugs (antihypertensive, statins, low-dose aspirin, beta-blockers). Patients with CAD and periodontitis + CAD presented lower serum retinol, α-carotene, β-carotene, γ-tocopherol, β-cryptoxanthin, lutein, zeaxanthin, and lycopene levels compared to periodontitis and healthy controls (Table 1).

Table 2 shows dental variables in patients with periodontitis, CAD, periodontitis + CAD, and controls. Patients with periodontitis and with periodontitis + CAD presented a lower median number of teeth and higher median values of periodontal parameters (CAL, PD, BOP, PI) compared with CAD and control subjects ($p < 0.001$). Moreover, the median values of periodontal parameters were significantly higher in patients in the periodontitis and periodontitis + CAD groups compared to patients with CAD and healthy controls ($p < 0.001$, Kruskal–Wallis test) (Table 2).

Table 1. Individual characteristics and biochemical parameters of recruited subjects.

	Controls (N = 36)	Periodontiti (N = 36)	CAD (N = 35)	Periodontitis + CAD (N = 36)
Age (years)	54 (51; 56)	55 (51; 57)	54 (48; 57)	55 (50; 56)
Gender (male/female)	17/19	18/18	19/17	17/19
Education level				
Primary school, n (%)	13 (36.1)	12 (33.3)	11 (31.4)	13 (36.1)
High school, n (%)	12 (33.3)	14 (38.9)	13 (37.1)	13 (36.1)
College/university, n (%)	11 (30.5)	10 (27.8)	11 (31.4)	10 (27.8)
Body mass index (kg/m^2)	25.6 (21.9; 27.7)	25.1 (22.8; 26.7)	25.9 (21.8; 28.4)	25.5 (21.7; 27.1)
Fasting glucose (mg/dL)	93.5 (87.7; 97.9)	94.4 (84.3; 106.2)	92.6 (87.9; 109.1)	93.1 (88.7; 111.2)
Current smokers, n (%)	3 (8.3)	3 (8.3)	2 (5.7)	3 (8.3)
Comorbidities				
Diabetes, n (%)		2 (14.2) **	3 (8.6) **	3 (8.3) **
Previous CVD				
Atrial fibrillation, n (%)			7 (20) **,§§	10 (27.8) **,§§
Angina pectoris, n (%)			16 (45.7) **,§§	17 (48.6) **,§§
Stroke, n (%)			7 (20) *,§§	9 (25.7) **,§§
Heart failure, n (%)			9 (25.7) **,§§	10 (27.8) **,§§
Drug treatment of CVD				
Antihypertensive, n (%)			13 (37.1) **,§§	14 (38.9) **,§§
Statins, n (%)			9 (25.7) **,§§	10 (27.8) **,§§
Low-dose aspirin, n (%)			9 (25.7) **,§§	11 (30.5) **,§§
Beta blockers, n (%)			10 (28.5) **,§§	12 (33.3) **,§§
hs-CRP (mg/L)	2.8 (2.2; 3.1)	3.7 (2.9; 4.2) *	6.4 (5.1; 6.9) **	6.8 (5.9; 7.7) **,§§,#
Total cholesterol (mg/dL)	174 (131; 189)	178 (152; 194)	181 (155; 197) *,§§	180 (149; 200)
Triglycerides (mg/dL)	130 (111; 144)	131 (57; 151)	134 (109; 157) *,§§	136 (117; 161)
Retinol (μmol/L)	2.12 (1.75; 2.47)	2.08 (1.89; 2.09)	2.05 (1.81; 2.07) *,§§	2.04 (1.78; 2.15) *,§§
α-carotene (μmol/L)	0.081 (0.051;0.123)	0.075 (0.041; 0.101)	0.073 (0.051; 0.123) *,§§	0.071 (0.049; 0.112) *,§§
β-carotene (μmol/L)	0.321 (0.22; 0.367)	0.317 (0.209; 0.361)	0.311 (0.278; 0.302) *,§§	0.309 (0.214; 0.355) *,§§
β-cryptoxanthin (μmol/L)	0.066 (0.043; 0.78)	0.059 (0.033; 0.71)	0.051 (0.029; 0.82) *,§§	0.048 (0.039; 0.64) *,§§
γ-tocopherol (μmol/L)	2.66 (2.35; 2.99)	2.63 (2.21; 2.73)	2.59 (2.12; 2.85) *,§§	2.57 (2.04; 2.78) *,§§
Lutein (μmol/L)	0.16 (0.11; 0.26)	0.14 (0.1; 0.19)	0.12 (0.08; 0.18) *,§§	0.11 (0.09; 0.21) *,§§
Zeaxanthin (μmol/L)	0.037 (0.024; 0.045)	0.034 (0.018; 0.039)	0.029 (0.021; 0.027) *,§§	0.031 (0.021; 0.042) *,§§
Lycopene (μmol/L)	0.36 (0.21; 0.42)	0.35 (0.22; 0.41)	0.32 (0.21; 0.39) *,§§	0.31 (0.19; 0.36) *

Data are expressed as median (25th and 75th percentiles) or number with percentage. * $p < 0.001$ and ** $p < 0.001$ significant differences vs. healthy subjects calculated by the Mann–Whitney test. §§ $p < 0.001$ significant differences vs. periodontitis patients calculated by the Mann–Whitney test. # $p < 0.008$ significant differences vs. CAD patients calculated by the Mann–Whitney test. CAD, ischemic heart disease; CVD, cardiovascular disease; hs-CRP, C-reactive protein.

Table 2. Clinical dental variables of recruited subjects.

	Controls (N = 36)	Periodontitis (N = 36)	CAD (N = 35)	Periodontitis + CAD (N = 36)
N of teeth	26 (24; 28)	19 (17; 20) **	23 (20; 24) **,§§	18 (13; 20) **,##
CAL (mm)	1.1 (0.8; 1.3)	4 (3.5; 4.2) **	2.1 (1.7; 2.4) **,§§	4.1 (3.6; 4.8) **,##
CAL 4–5 mm (% sites)		38.7 (36.2; 43.4) **		42.2 (38.9; 48.7) **,##
CAL ≥6 mm (% sites)		20.2 (16.8; 21.7) **		18.2 (16.4; 24.2) **,##
PD (mm)	1.4 (1.1; 1.8)	4.5 (4.1; 5.2) **	2 (1.9; 2.3) **,§§	4.1 (3.8; 4.7) **,##
PD 4–5 mm (% sites)		42.1 (40.1; 46.4) **		44.8 (41.5; 51.1) **,##
PD ≥6 mm (% sites)		22.3 (17.9; 23.1) **		23.9 (21.6; 27.6) **,§§,##
BOP (%)	8.8 (6.1; 10.9)	47.1 (45.1; 48.9) **	8.7 (5.2; 9.2) **,§§	45.7 (44.6; 56.2) **,§§,##
PI (%)	6.9 (5.3; 10.8)	34.9 (33.3; 36.1) **	12.9 (12.1; 13.4) **,§§	34.3 (31.2; 35.1) **,##

Data are expressed as median (25th and 75th percentile). ** $p < 0.001$ significant differences vs. control subjects calculated by the Mann–Whitney test. §§ $p < 0.001$ significant differences vs. periodontitis patients calculated by the Mann–Whitney test. ## $p < 0.001$ significant differences vs. CAD patients calculated by the Mann–Whitney test. CAL, clinical attachment level; PD, probing pocket depth; BOP, bleeding on probing; PI, plaque index.

vitamin C Evaluation

Median (25th and 75th percentile) serum and salivary vitamin C levels are presented in Figure 2. The median concentrations of serum and salivary vitamin C were lower in the CAD ($p < 0.01$) and in the periodontitis + CAD ($p < 0.001$) groups compared to controls. Serum and salivary vitamin C concentrations were also significantly decreased in patients of the periodontitis + CAD group in comparison with periodontitis patients ($p < 0.01$; Figure 2). Overall, the p-value for trend analysis performed (Jonckheere–Terpstra test) indicated that serum vitamin C progressively decreased in patients with periodontitis, CAD, and periodontitis + CAD ($p < 0.001$; Figure 2).

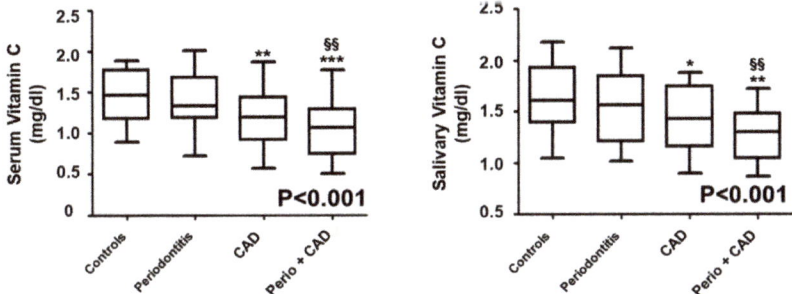

Figure 2. Median values (25% and 75% percentiles) of serum and salivary vitamin C levels in each group of subjects. * $p < 0.05$, ** $p < 0.01$, and *** $p < 0.001$ significant differences vs. control subjects (derived by Kruskal–Wallis test). §§ $p < 0.01$ significant differences vs. periodontitis patients. $p < 0.001$ (obtained by Jonckheere–Terpstra test).

There was no statistically significant correlation between salivary and serum vitamin C levels (rs = 0.157, $p = 0.087$; Figure 3).

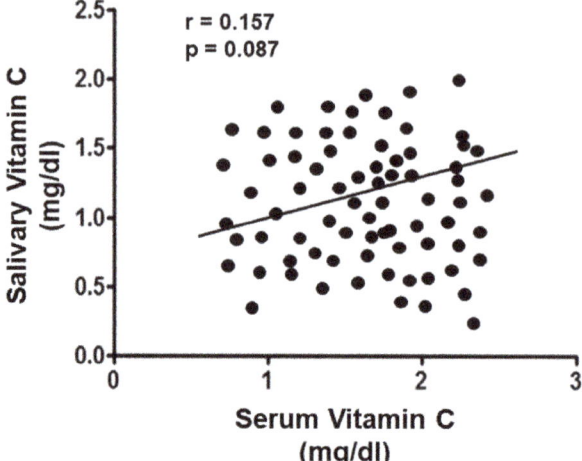

Figure 3. Correlation analysis of serum and salivary vitamin C levels in all enrolled subjects.

Moreover, across all subjects, serum/salivary vitamin C concentrations correlated negatively (rs = −0.378, $p < 0.001$)/(rs = −0.427, $p < 0.001$) with hs-CRP levels (Figure 4).

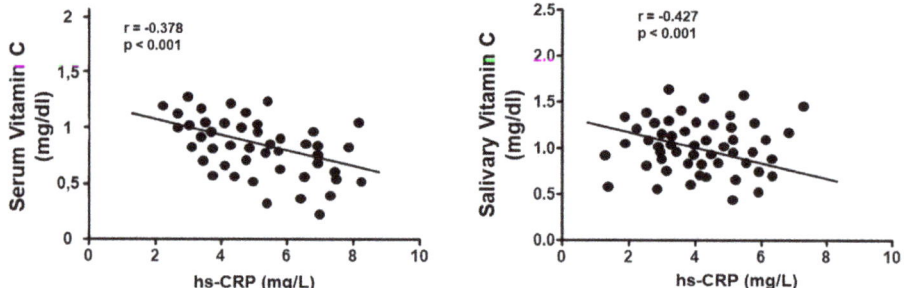

Figure 4. Correlation analysis of serum and salivary vitamin C levels with CRP values in all enrolled subjects.

The adjusted multivariate linear regression analysis, aimed at assessing the possible association of periodontitis and CAD on serum and salivary vitamin C levels, showed that hs-CRP ($p < 0.001$) was the only statistically significant predictor variable for serum vitamin C; hs-CRP ($p < 0.001$) and triglycerides ($p = 0.028$) were the statistically significant predictor variables for salivary vitamin C (Table 3).

Table 3. Uni- and multivariate linear regression model for serum and salivary vitamin C levels in all enrolled subjects.

Variable	Univariate			Multivariate		
	B	95% CI	p	B	95% CI	p
Serum vitamin C levels						
CAD	−0.378	−0.222; 0.578	<0.001	−0.069	−0.341; 0.498	0.644
Periodontitis	−0.223	−0.016; 0.404	0.034	−0.141	−0.039; 0.389	0.112
hs-CRP	−0.119	−0.075; 0.137	<0.001	−0.112	0.065; 0.149	<0.001
Age (years)	0.078	0.29; 0.004	0.081	0.039	−0.148; 0.187	0.436
Female gender	−0.149	−0.041; 0.327	0.149	−0.178	−0.112; 0.344	0.078
Triglycerides	−0.066	−0.199; 0.078	0.209	0.074	−0.167; 0.366	0.141
Salivary vitamin C levels						
CAD	−0.236	0.134; 0.41	<0.001	−0.029	−0.433; 0.312	0.655
Periodontitis	−0.064	−0.087; 0.214	0.387	0.005	−0.151; 0.184	0.972
hs-CRP	−0.078	0.038; 0.132	<0.001	0.077	0.061; 0.146	<0.001
Age (years)	0.041	−0.041; 0.012	0.207	0.012	−0.029; 0.036	0.786
Female gender	−0.038	−0.114; 0.226	0.419	0.079	−0.047; 0.239	0.178
Triglycerides	0.079	−0.178; 0.006	0.039	−0.714	−0.058; 0.241	0.028
Serum vitamin C	−0.149	−0.031; 0.378	0.079	−0.029	−0.223; 0.154	0.599

Age was included as a continuous variable. For periodontitis and CAD, controls served as reference. For gender, males served as reference. For education, primary school served as a reference.

4. Discussion

This study evaluated the association of different conditions such as gingival health, periodontitis, CAD, or a combination of both diseases (periodontitis and CAD) on saliva and serum vitamin C levels. This study found that periodontitis in CAD patients was associated with decreased levels of serum and salivary vitamin C and hs-CRP levels. However, compared to periodontitis and healthy subjects, only patients with CAD and periodontitis + CAD presented significantly lower salivary and serum vitamin C levels, supporting the hypothesis that CAD may have contributed to decreased serum and salivary vitamin C levels.

Moreover, our results showed that the presence of periodontitis in patients with CAD might serve as an inhibitor of vitamin C and for associated risk of CAD and CVD. Recent investigations suggested that low serum vitamin C levels, through inactivation of NO signaling, are independent risk factors of CVD and related to increased mortality [32]. More specifically, it has also been demonstrated that a decrease in vitamin C levels was associated with carotid endothelial damage in patients with atherosclerosis, highlighting the positive role of vitamin C and antioxidants on NO levels [33]. The co-occurrence of periodontitis in CAD patients may be a possible pathway for the observed deterioration of endothelial function via decreased vitamin C levels. Periodontal treatment clinically decreased serum vitamin C and antioxidants levels in patients with chronic kidney disease [34].

As a support of the present study, several lines of evidence have shown that stimulating oxidative stress conditions, such as periodontitis and CAD, may have led to the lower the production of vitamin C, which in turn could augment serum and salivary CRP levels [35]. The high inflammation present during periodontitis and CAD is believed to accelerate vitamin C oxidation [35]. In accordance with our results, Amaliya et al. [36] found that low serum vitamin C and high CRP levels were associated in a dose-dependent manner in a sample of 98 subjects with periodontitis.

Moreover, while there are some observations on the serum vitamin C levels as a marker for endothelial dysfunction or CAD risk, there are no reports that analyze both salivary and serum vitamin C levels during periodontitis. However, the present study did not find a statistically significant correlation between serum and salivary vitamin C levels; salivary vitamin C levels were associated by hs-CRP levels. This could be explained by the fact that the saliva levels of vitamin C could mainly reflect the serum vitamin C levels or that the salivary vitamin C levels may have been influenced by the saliva collection method used in the present study [37].

In the present study, patients with CAD and with periodontitis plus CAD presented low salivary vitamin C levels, in accordance with previous studies which demonstrated that saliva contains many biochemical systems known to be involved in soft-tissue repair, and many antibacterial components, including lysozyme, lactoferrin, and salivary peroxidase [38]. Human whole saliva contains a complex peroxidase system, the major components of which include different forms of lactoperoxidase secreted by the salivary glands and myeloperoxidases from polymorphonucleocytes [39].

While the systemic impact of reduced vitamin C levels on endothelial dysfunction via decreased NO has been demonstrated, the effect of oral vitamin C is less clear. As a matter of fact, there are reports which show that periodontitis is positively associated with impaired salivary NO levels [19,24]. NO can be produced in the gingival tissues as part of the oral unspecific salivary antibacterial defense against anaerobic periodontopathogens bacteria [12,24,40]. In this regard, some reports showed high levels of NO synthesis and activity in the inflamed periodontal tissue [25,41–44]. Another explanation for the contradictory results may be due to the method of saliva collection. Moreover, it can also be argued that the difference in NO production at the periodontal level is probably different from NO in the bloodstream: In the mouth, it is an antibacterial defense, whereas systemically, it impacts endothelial function.

Moreover, endothelial dysfunctions in periodontitis patients with CAD could be due to a specific immunoreactive pathway in which vitamin C modulates an anti-inflammatory response against periodontopathic bacteria during periodontitis. It has been shown that vitamin C, during periodontitis is involved in immune response through the activated endothelium and its heat shock proteins that are present in the endothelium surface, finally stimulating some cross-reactive T-cells with particularity for host-activated antibodies [45,46]. This process, modulated by vitamin C, also affects the inducted defense mechanism mediated by NO, which promotes the hyperactivation of the endothelial cells that increases the risk of further infection or systemic inflammation due to periodontitis [47–49].

However, the present preliminary study presents some limitations. One of the main limitations is the cross-sectional nature of the study, which does not allow any evaluation on the impact of vitamin C levels on periodontitis, which should be assessed only with a longitudinal observation. Another limitation is the small sample size, which was due to matching age, gender, and education. An advantage of matching is the elimination of the impact of these confounding variables. Significant limitations also include the lack of analysis for dietary quality (e.g., intake of vitamin C and statins) and the analysis of alpha-tocopherol.

5. Conclusions

During the last few decades, new approaches through salivary diagnostics have been developed to evaluate the possible useful biomarkers for predicting the disease. This study indicated that patients who have periodontitis and CAD presented lower serum and salivary vitamin C and antioxidant levels compared to patients with periodontitis and healthy subjects. Moreover, this study suggests that mainly CAD acts as a key factor on serum and salivary vitamin C and antioxidant levels through a pathway mediated by the CRP. This pilot study is promising and demands further studies with a larger sample and longitudinal observation in saliva, serum, and gingival crevicular fluid in order to better understand the role of vitamin C levels during periodontitis.

Supplementary Materials: The following are available online at http://www.mdpi.com/2072-6643/11/12/2956/s1: Table S1. STROBE Statement—checklist of items that should be included in reports of observational studies.

Author Contributions: G.I. conceived the idea and wrote the paper. G.I., A.P., S.M., and A.L.G. reviewed the collected data. G.I. and R.L. were responsible for editing, original data, and text preparation. All authors took responsibility for the integrity of the data that is present in this study.

Funding: This research received no external funding.

Conflicts of Interest: The authors declare no conflict of interest.

References

1. Eke, P.I.; Wei, L.; Thornton-Evans, G.O.; Borrell, L.N.; Borgnakke, W.S.; Dye, B.; Genco, R.J. Risk Indicators for Periodontitis in US Adults: NHANES 2009 to 2012. *J. Periodontol.* **2016**, *87*, 1174–1185. [CrossRef] [PubMed]
2. Isola, G.; Polizzi, A.; Santonocito, S.; Alibrandi, A.; Ferlito, S. Expression of Salivary And Serum Malondialdehyde And Lipid Profile Of Patients With Periodontitis And Coronary Heart Disease. *Int. J. Mol. Sci.* **2019**, *20*, 6061. [CrossRef]
3. Bernabe, E.; Dahiya, M.; Bhandari, B.; Murray, C.J.; Marcenes, W. Global burden of severe periodontitis in 1990–2010: A systematic review and meta-regression. *J. Dent. Res.* **2014**, *93*, 1045–1053.
4. Friedewald, V.E.; Kornman, K.S.; Beck, J.D.; Genco, R.; Goldfine, A.; Libby, P.; Offenbacher, S.; Ridker, P.M.; Van Dyke, T.E.; Roberts, W.C. American Journal of Cardiology; Journal of Periodontology. The American Journal of Cardiology and Journal of Periodontology editors' consensus: Periodontitis and atherosclerotic cardiovascular disease. *J. Periodontol.* **2009**, *80*, 1021–1032. [CrossRef] [PubMed]
5. Seymour, G.J.; Palmer, J.E.; Leishman, S.J.; Do, H.L.; Westerman, B.; Carle, A.D.; Faddy, M.J.; West, M.J.; Cullinan, M.P. Influence of a triclosan toothpaste on periodontopathic bacteria and periodontitis progression in cardiovascular patients: A randomized controlled trial. *J. Periodontal Res.* **2017**, *52*, 61–73. [CrossRef]
6. Holmlund, A.; Holm, G.; Lind, L. Number of teeth as a predictor of cardiovascular mortality in a cohort of 7,674 subjects followed for 12 years. *J. Periodontol.* **2010**, *81*, 870–876. [CrossRef]
7. Isola, G.; Alibrandi, A.; Currò, M.; Matarese, M.; Ricca, S.; Matarese, G.; Kocher, T. Evaluation of salivary and serum ADMA levels in patients with periodontal and cardiovascular disease as subclinical marker of cardiovascular risk. *J. Periodontol* **2019**, in press.
8. Isola, G.; Matarese, G.; Ramaglia, L.; Pedullà, E.; Rapisarda, E.; Iorio-Siciliano, V. Association between periodontitis and glycosylated hemoglobin before diabetes onset: A cross-sectional study. *Clin. Oral Investig.* **2019**. [CrossRef]
9. Vidal, F.; Figueredo, C.M.; Cordovil, I.; Fischer, R.G. Periodontal therapy reduces plasma levels of interleukin-6, C-reactive protein, and fibrinogen in patients with severe periodontitis and refractory arterial hypertension. *J. Periodontol.* **2009**, *80*, 786–791. [CrossRef]
10. Isola, G.; Lo Giudice, A.; Polizzi, A.; Alibrandi, A.; Patini, R.; Ferlito, S. Association of Circulating Progenitor Cells Levels during Periodontitis. *Genes* **2019**, in press.
11. Tyml, K. vitamin C and Microvascular Dysfunction in Systemic Inflammation. *Antioxidants (Basel)* **2017**, *6*, 49. [CrossRef] [PubMed]
12. Hampton, T.G.; Amende, I.; Fong, J.; Laubach, V.E.; Li, J.; Metais, C.; Simons, M. Basic FGF reduces stunning via a NOS2-dependent pathway in coronary perfused mouse hearts. *Am. J. Physiol. Heart Circ. Physiol.* **2000**, *279*, H260–H268. [CrossRef] [PubMed]
13. Engler, M.M.; Engler, M.B.; Malloy, M.J.; Chiu, E.Y.; Schloetter, M.C.; Paul, S.M.; Stuehlinger, M.; Lin, K.Y.; Cooke, J.P.; Morrow, J.D.; et al. Antioxidant vitamins C and E improve endothelial function in children with hyperlipidemia: Endothelial Assessment of Risk from Lipids in Youth (EARLY) Trial. *Circulation* **2003**, *108*, 1059–1063. [CrossRef] [PubMed]
14. Song, E.K.; Kang, S.M. vitamin C Deficiency, High-Sensitivity C-Reactive Protein, and Cardiac Event-Free Survival in Patients with Heart Failure. *J. Cardiovasc. Nurs.* **2018**, *33*, 6–12. [CrossRef] [PubMed]
15. Rodrigo, R.; Hasson, D.; Prieto, J.C.; Dussaillant, G.; Ramos, C.; León, L.; Gárate, J.; Valls, N.; Gormaz, J.G. The effectiveness of antioxidant vitamins C and E in reducing myocardial infarct size in patients subjected to percutaneous coronary angioplasty (PREVEC Trial): Study protocol for a pilot randomized double-blind controlled trial. *Trials* **2014**, *15*, 192. [CrossRef] [PubMed]
16. Isola, G.; Alibrandi, A.; Rapisarda, E.; Matarese, G.; Williams, R.C.; Leonardi, R. Association of vitamin d in patients with periodontal and cardiovascular disease: A cross-sectional study. *J. Periodontal Res.* **2019**, in press.
17. Tonetti, M.S.; D'Aiuto, F.; Nibali, L.; Donald, A.; Storry, C.; Parkar, M.; Suvan, J.; Hingorani, A.D.; Vallance, P.; Deanfield, J. Treatment of periodontitis and endothelial function. *New Engl. J. Med.* **2007**, *356*, 911–920. [CrossRef]
18. Holtfreter, B.; Empen, K.; Glaser, S.; Gläser, S.; Lorbeer, R.; Völzke, H.; Ewert, R.; Kocher, T.; Dörr, M. Periodontitis is associated with endothelial dysfunction in a general population: A cross-sectional study. *PLoS ONE* **2013**, *8*, e84603. [CrossRef]

19. Andrukhov, O.; Haririan, H.; Bertl, K.; Rausch, W.D.; Bantleon, H.P.; Moritz, A.; Rausch-Fan, X. Nitric oxide production, systemic inflammation and lipid metabolism in periodontitis patients: Possible gender aspect. *J. Clin. Periodontol.* **2013**, *40*, 916–923. [CrossRef]
20. Huang, A.L.; Vita, J.A. Effects of systemic inflammation on endothelium-dependent vasodilation. *Trends Cardiovasc. Med.* **2006**, *16*, 15–20. [CrossRef]
21. Gurav, A.N. The implication of periodontitis in vascular endothelial dysfunction. *Eur. J. Clin. Investig.* **2014**, *44*, 1000–1009. [CrossRef] [PubMed]
22. Mah, E.; Matos, M.D.; Kawiecki, D.; Ballard, K.; Guo, Y.; Volek, J.S.; Bruno, R.S. vitamin C status is related to proinflammatory responses and impaired vascular endothelial function in healthy, college-aged lean and obese men. *J. Am. Diet. Assoc.* **2011**, *111*, 737–743. [CrossRef] [PubMed]
23. Nishida, M.; Grossi, S.G.; Dunford, R.G.; Ho, A.W.; Trevisan, M.; Genco, R.J. Dietary vitamin C and the risk for periodontal disease. *J. Periodontol.* **2000**, *71*, 1215–1223. [CrossRef] [PubMed]
24. Kendall, H.K.; Marshall, R.I.; Bartold, P.M. Nitric oxide and tissue destruction. *Oral Dis.* **2001**, *7*, 2–10. [CrossRef] [PubMed]
25. Amarasena, N.; Ogawa, H.; Yoshihara, A.; Hanada, N.; Miyazaki, H. Serum vitamin C-periodontal relationship in community-dwelling elderly Japanese. *J. Clin. Periodontol.* **2005**, *32*, 93–97. [CrossRef]
26. Harej, A.; Macan, A.M.; Stepanić, V.; Klobučar, M.; Pavelić, K.; Pavelić, S.K.; Raić-Malić, S. The Antioxidant and Antiproliferative Activities of 1,2,3-Triazolyl-L-Ascorbic Acid Derivatives. *Int. J. Mol. Sci.* **2019**, *20*, 4735. [CrossRef]
27. von Elm, E.; Altman, D.G.; Egger, M.; Pocock, S.J.; Gotzsche, P.C.; Vandenbroucke, J.P. The Strengthening the Reporting ofObservational Studies in Epidemiology (STROBE) statement: Guidelines for reporting observational studies. *J. Clin. Periodontol.* **2008**, *61*, 344–349.
28. Tonetti, M.S.; Greenwell, H.; Kornman, K.S. Staging and grading of periodontitis: Framework and proposal of a new classification and case definition. *J. Periodontol.* **2018**, *89*, S159–S172. [CrossRef]
29. Isola, G.; Matarese, M.; Ramaglia, L.; Iorio-Siciliano, V.; Cordasco, G.; Matarese, G. Efficacy of a drug composed of herbal extracts on postoperative discomfort after surgical removal of impacted mandibular third molar: A randomized, triple-blind, controlled clinical trial. *Clin. Oral Investig.* **2019**, *23*, 2443–2453. [CrossRef]
30. Bassand, J.P.; Hamm, C.W.; Ardissino, D.; Boersma, E.; Budaj, A.; Fernandez-Aviles, F.; Fox, K.A.; Hasdai, D.; Ohman, E.M.; Wallentin, L.; et al. Guidelines for the diagnosis and treatment of non-ST-segment elevation acute coronary syndromes: The Task Force for the Diagnosis and Treatment of Non-ST-Segment Elevation Acute Coronary Syndromes of the European Society of Cardiology. *Eur. Heart J.* **2007**, *28*, 1598–1660. [CrossRef]
31. O'Leary, T.J.; Drake, R.B.; Naylor, J.E. The plaque control record. *J. Periodontol.* **1972**, *43*, 38. [CrossRef] [PubMed]
32. Aune, D.; Keum, N.; Giovannucci, E.; Fadnes, L.T.; Boffetta, P.; Greenwood, D.C.; Tonstad, S.; Vatten, L.J.; Riboli, E.; Norat, T. Dietary intake and blood concentrations of antioxidants and the risk of cardiovascular disease, total cancer, and all-cause mortality: A systematic review and dose-response meta-analysis of prospective studies. *Am. J. Clin. Nutr.* **2018**, *108*, 1069–1091. [CrossRef] [PubMed]
33. Polidori, M.C.; Ruggiero, C.; Croce, M.F.; Raichi, T.; Mangialasche, F.; Cecchetti, R.; Pelini, L.; Paolacci, L.; Ercolani, S.; Mecocci, P. Association of increased carotid intima-media thickness and lower plasma levels of vitamin C and vitamin E in old age subjects: Implications for Alzheimer's disease. *J. Neural. Transm. (Vienna)* **2015**, *122*, 523–530. [CrossRef] [PubMed]
34. Mathias, T.M.; Silva, J.F.; Sapata, V.M.; Marson, F.C.; Zanoni, J.N.; Silva, C.O. Evaluation of the effects of periodontal treatment on levels of ascorbic acid in smokers. *J. Int. Acad. Periodontol.* **2014**, *16*, 109–114. [PubMed]
35. Ellulu, M.S.; Rahmat, A.; Patimah, I.; Khaza'ai, H.; Abed, Y. Effect of vitamin C on inflammation and metabolic markers in hypertensive and/or diabetic obese adults: A randomized controlled trial. *Drug Des. Dev. Ther.* **2015**, *9*, 3405–3412. [CrossRef] [PubMed]
36. Amaliya, A.; Laine, M.L.; Loos, B.G.; Van der Velden, U. Java project on periodontal diseases: Effect of vitamin C/calcium threonate/citrus flavonoids supplementation on periodontal pathogens, CRP and HbA1c. *J. Clin. Periodontol.* **2015**, *42*, 1097–1104. [CrossRef]

37. Golatowski, C.; Salazar, M.G.; Dhople, V.M.; Hammer, E.; Kocher, T.; Jehmlich, N.; Völker, U. Comparative evaluation of saliva collection methods for proteome analysis. *Clin. Chim. Acta* **2013**, *419*, 42–46. [CrossRef]
38. Rice-Evans, C.; Miller, N.J. Total antioxidant status in plasma and body fluids. *Methods Enzymol.* **1994**, *234*, 279–293.
39. Battino, M.; Ferreiro, M.S.; Gallardo, I.; Newman, H.N.; Bullon, P. The antioxidant capacity of saliva. *J. Clin. Periodontol.* **2002**, *29*, 189–194. [CrossRef]
40. Rausch-Fan, X.; Matejka, M. From plaque formation to periodontal disease, is there a role for nitric oxide? *Eur. J. Clin. Investig.* **2001**, *31*, 833–835. [CrossRef]
41. Matejka, M.; Patyka, L.; Ulm, C.; Solar, P.; Sinzinger, H. Nitric oxide synthesis is increased in periodontal disease. *J. Period. Res.* **1998**, *33*, 517–518. [CrossRef] [PubMed]
42. Gullu, C.; Ozmeric, N.; Tokman, B.; Elgun, S.; Balos, K. Effectiveness of scaling and root planing versus modified Widman flap on nitric oxide synthase and arginase activity in patients with chronic periodontitis. *J. Period. Res.* **2005**, *40*, 168–175. [CrossRef] [PubMed]
43. Ozer, L.; Elgun, S.; Ozdemir, B.; Pervane, B.; Ozmeric, N. Arginine-nitric oxide-polyamine metabolism in periodontal disease. *J. Periodontol.* **2011**, *82*, 320–328. [CrossRef] [PubMed]
44. Patini, R.; Staderini, E.; Gallenzi, P. Multidisciplinary surgical management of Cowden syndrome: Report of a case. *J. Clin. Exp. Dent.* **2016**, *8*, e472–e474. [CrossRef] [PubMed]
45. Ekuni, D.; Tomofuji, T.; Sanbe, T.; Irie, K.; Azuma, T.; Maruyama, T.; Tamaki, N.; Murakami, J.; Kokeguchi, S.; Yamamoto, T. vitamin C intake attenuates the degree of experimental atherosclerosis induced by periodontitis in the rat by decreasing oxidative stress. *Arch. Oral Biol.* **2009**, *54*, 495–502. [CrossRef]
46. Kaur, G.; Kathariya, R.; Bansal, S.; Singh, A.; Shahakar, D. Dietary antioxidants and their indispensable role in periodontal health. *J. Food Drug Anal.* **2016**, *24*, 239–246. [CrossRef]
47. Caccianiga, G.; Paiusco, A.; Perillo, L.; Nucera, R.; Pinsino, A.; Maddalone, M.; Cordasco, G.; Lo Giudice, A. Does low-level laser therapy enhance the efficiency of orthodontic dental alignment? Results from a randomized pilot study. *Photomed. Laser Surg.* **2017**, *35*, 421–426. [CrossRef]
48. Caccianiga, G.; Crestale, C.; Cozzani, M.; Piras, A.; Mutinelli, S.; Lo Giudice, A., Cordasco, G. Low-level laser therapy and invisible removal aligners. *J. Biol. Regul. Homeost. Agents* **2016**, *30*, 107–113.
49. Takahama, U.; Hirota, S.; Oniki, T. Quercetin-dependent scavenging of reactive nitrogen species derived from nitric oxide and nitrite in the human oral cavity: Interaction of quercetin with salivary redox components. *Arch. Oral Biol.* **2006**, *51*, 629–639. [CrossRef]

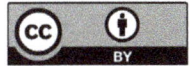

© 2019 by the authors. Licensee MDPI, Basel, Switzerland. This article is an open access article distributed under the terms and conditions of the Creative Commons Attribution (CC BY) license (http://creativecommons.org/licenses/by/4.0/).

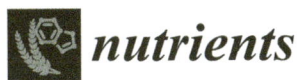

Article

Investigation of Antibacterial and Antiinflammatory Activities of Proanthocyanidins from *Pelargonium sidoides* DC Root Extract

Aiste Jekabsone [1,*], Inga Sile [2,3], Andrea Cochis [4,5], Marina Makrecka-Kuka [2,3], Goda Laucaityte [1], Elina Makarova [2], Lia Rimondini [4,5], Rasa Bernotiene [1], Lina Raudone [1], Evelina Vedlugaite [6], Rasa Baniene [1], Alina Smalinskiene [1], Nijole Savickiene [1] and Maija Dambrova [2,3]

1. Medical Academy, Lithuanian University of Health Sciences, Sukileliu Ave. 13, LT-50162 Kaunas, Lithuania
2. Latvian Institute of Organic Synthesis, Aizkraukles Str. 21, LV1006 Riga, Latvia
3. Riga Stradins University, Dzirciema Str. 16, LV1007, Latvia
4. Department of Health Sciences, University of Piemonte Orientale, Via Solaroli 17, 28100 Novara, Italy
5. Interdisciplinary Research Center of Autoimmune Diseases, Center for Translational Research on Autoimmune and Allergic Diseases–CAAD, C.so Trieste 15A, 28100 Novara, Italy
6. Clinic of dental and oral pathology, LSMU Hospital, Kaunas Clinics, Medical academy, Lithuanian University of Health Sciences, Eiveniu Str. 2, LT-50161 Kaunas, Lithuania
* Correspondence: aiste.jekabsone@lsmuni.lt; Tel.: +370-675-94455

Received: 16 September 2019; Accepted: 8 November 2019; Published: 19 November 2019

Abstract: The study explores antibacterial, antiinflammatory and cytoprotective capacity of *Pelargonium sidoides* DC root extract (PSRE) and proanthocyanidin fraction from PSRE (PACN) under conditions characteristic for periodontal disease. Following previous finding that PACN exerts stronger suppression of *Porphyromonas gingivalis* compared to the effect on commensal *Streptococcus salivarius*, the current work continues antibacterial investigation on *Staphylococcus aureus*, *Staphylococcus epidermidis*, *Aggregatibacter actinomycetemcomitans* and *Escherichia coli*. PSRE and PACN are also studied for their ability to prevent gingival fibroblast cell death in the presence of bacteria or bacterial lipopolysaccharide (LPS), to block LPS- or LPS + IFNγ-induced release of inflammatory mediators, gene expression and surface antigen presentation. Both PSRE and PACN were more efficient in suppressing *Staphylococcus* and *Aggregatibacter* compared to *Escherichia*, prevented *A. actinomycetemcomitans*- and LPS-induced death of fibroblasts, decreased LPS-induced release of interleukin-8 and prostaglandin E2 from fibroblasts and IL-6 from leukocytes, blocked expression of IL-1β, iNOS, and surface presentation of CD80 and CD86 in LPS + IFNγ-treated macrophages, and IL-1β and COX-2 expression in LPS-treated leukocytes. None of the investigated substances affected either the level of secretion or expression of TNFα. In conclusion, PSRE, and especially PACN, possess strong antibacterial, antiinflammatory and gingival tissue protecting properties under periodontitis-mimicking conditions and are suggestable candidates for treatment of the disease.

Keywords: periodontitis; *Pelargonium sidoides* DC root extract; proanthocyanidins; bacteriotoxicity; inflammatory cytokines; gene expression; fibroblasts; macrophages; leukocytes

1. Introduction

Periodontitis is an infectious inflammatory disease resulting in periodontal pocket formation, progressive bone reduction and teeth loss in many industrialized countries [1,2]. Common treatment strategies include systemic use of antibiotics and local synthetic antiseptic substances, both leading to undesirable side effects and increased resistance of bacteria [3]. In consequence, prolonged and/or repeatable treatment is risky, inefficient and fails to stop disease remission and further progression. In fact, as a response to the extensive use of drugs, bacteria have developed a new mechanism to skip and counteract antibiotics activity: resistant polysaccharide envelope, more efficient efflux pumps, intracellular modifications and genetic mutations are some of the pathways exploited by bacteria to withstand drugs effect [4]. However, it is important to consider that not all body-resident bacteria are pathogens: commensal strain present in the microbiota play a pivotal role in preserving homeostasis in the skin and mucosal physiological systems of the human body [5,6]. The use of very strong chemicals such as chlorhexidine [7] can be exploited only for short periods to prevent severe side effects that can occur after prolonged exposure [8]. It follows that an ideal new antibacterial compound should be able to affect bacteria metabolism by a different mechanism than those exploited by antibiotics but at the same time would be harmless to the healthy cells and commensal bacteria. In this light, multicomponent plant-derived antibacterial substances like proanthocyanidins (PACN) make a promising alternative and adjunctive therapy candidates for periodontitis treatment because of a lower risk of resistance development and side effects [9].

PACN are condensed tannins constructed form flavan-3-ol units [10]. The compounds possess a range of biological activities including anti-inflammatory and antibacterial [11]. The capacity of PACN to suppress inflammation is related to both strong antioxidant and metalloproteinase (MMP) inhibiting properties [12,13], whereas antibacterial efficiency is achieved due to prevention of bacterial adhesion and biofilm formation [14]. The chemical nature of PACN in crude extracts varies depending on plant species used. *Pelargonium sidoides* DC, a medicinal plant native to South Africa, is one of the most PACN-enriched plants. Medicinal raw materials—roots of the plant—are used in the treatment of infectious and inflammatory disorders, and *P. sidoides* root extracts (PSREs) possess the same properties with enhanced efficiency [15–18]. PSREs mediate their pharmacological effects via two classes of compounds, namely oxygenated coumarins and prodelphinidins that belong to the PACN group [18]. The common properties of these compounds isolated from various sources suggest the significant part of the activities of PSREs might be assigned to PACN. Indeed, we have recently shown that namely prodelphinidin fraction from PSRE more efficiently suppress periodontal pathogens *Porphyromonas gingivalis* compared to PSRE itself [19]. Moreover, the activity appeared to be strain selective: reducing the viability of the pathogens while preserving the metabolic activity of the beneficial oral commensal *Streptococcus salivarius*.

Based on these promising results, in the present study we decided to extend the examination of antibacterial efficiency of PACN to other broad-range pathogens and commensals: two commercial drug-resistant *Staphylococcus aureus* and *Aggregatibacter actinomycetemcomitans* strains, a clinical isolate pathogen *Staphylococcus epidermidis* strain and a commensal *Escherichia coli* strain. Next, after verifying extract cytocompatibility towards gingival fibroblasts, a "race for the surface" model of bacteria-cells co-culture [20] was carried out to verify the extract ability to reduce bacteria proliferation while preserving cells viability in the same microenvironment where cells and bacteria compete for the same surface. Finally, we have made an extensive investigation on PACN activity in bacterial lipopolysaccharide (LPS)-mediated inflammation, including measurement of secretion of inflammatory cytokines and other mediators, inflammatory gene expression and viability of gingival fibroblasts, macrophages and blood leukocytes.

2. Materials and Methods

2.1. Pelargonium sidoides Root Extract and Proanthocyanidin Fraction

The *P. sidoides* root extract (PSRE) was purchased from Frutarom Switzerland Ltd. Rutiwisstrasse 7 CH-8820 Wadenswil (batch no. 0410100). Proanthocyanidins (PACN) from PSRE were purified as described by Hellström and co-authors [21] with some modifications [19]. Briefly, 4 g of PSRE was dissolved in 200 mL of 50% methanol, the solution was centrifuged at 2000× g for 20 min and filtered through 0.45 µm nylon filters. The solution was purified by gel adsorption over Sephadex LH-20. The proanthocyanidins were released from the gel with 70% aqueous acetone (500 mL) and concentrated under vacuum at 35 °C. The aqueous aliquot was freeze-dried. The freeze dried PACN preparation yielded in 1.37 ± 0.07 g and comprised about 34.25% of the loaded PSRE.

2.2. Bacterial Strains and Growth Conditions

Commercially available strains *Staphylococcus aureus* (*S. aureus*, pathogen, ATCC 43300), *Aggregatibacter actinomycetemcomitans* (*A. actinomycetemcomitans*, pathogen, ATCC 33384) and *Escherichia coli* (*E. coli*, non-pathogen, ATCC BAA-1427) were purchased from the American Type Culture Collection (ATCC, MA, USA) and cultivated following the manufacturer's instructions. A clinical isolate of *Staphylococcus epidermidis* (*S. epidermidis*, pathogen) was collected at the Clinical Microbiology Unit at the Novara Maggiore Hospital (Novara, Italy). The clinical isolate was obtained after patient's informed consent in full accordance with the Declaration of Helsinki. Clinical strain was cultivated in Luria-Bertani medium (LB, Sigma-Aldrich, Milan, Italy) at 37 °C. For experiments, a single colony from each strain was collected and inoculated in 9 mL of LB broth at 37 °C overnight (18 h). After incubation, a new fresh LB tube diluted 1:10 was prepared and incubated at 37 °C for 3 h to achieve the logarithmic growth phase. Finally, broth cultures were diluted in LB broth until the optical density was 0.001 at 600 nm, corresponding to a final concentration of 1×10^5 cells/mL.

2.3. Antibacterial Efficiency Evaluation

To test antibacterial activity, PSRE and PACN were used at the following concentrations: 10, 30, 50, 70, 80, 90 and 100 µg/mL. PSRE and PACN powders were mixed and diluted directly into LB medium containing the desired bacteria concentration (described in 2.2. chapter); 1 mL of the obtained mix solutions (LB containing bacteria + PSRE/PACN) was seeded in the wells of a 24 multiwell plate (SPL, BioSigma, Milan, Italy) and incubated 24 h at 37 °C. Bacteria cultivated into pure LB medium were considered as control. After incubation, bacteria viability was evaluated by means of the colorimetric metabolic assay Alamar blue (alamarBlue®, Thermo-Fisher, Waltham, MA, USA) following the manufacturer's instructions. Briefly, the ready-to-use solution was added to each well in a 1:10 ratio and incubated for 4 h in the dark at 37 °C; then, fluorescence was recorded at 590 nm using a spectrophotometer (Spark, Tecan, Basel, Switzerland).

2.4. Co-Cultures of Human Gingival Fibroblasts and Bacteria

To verify PSRE and PACN ability to preserve cells metabolism in the presence of infection, a race for the surface cells-bacteria co-culture experiment was set up. *S. aureus* and *A. actinomycetemcomitans* were selected and used with cells to simulate the oral and mucosal environments, respectively. Human primary gingival fibroblasts (HGF, ATCC PCS-201-018) were used as a cellular model to be tested with bacteria. Cells were seeded at a defined number (1.5×10^4 cells/well) in the wells of a 24 multiwell plate and allowed to adhere overnight. Afterwards, the medium was removed and replaced by 1 mL of solution composed by an antibiotics-free medium (minimal essential medium Eagle alpha-modification, from Sigma) supplemented with 10% fetal bovine serum (FBS, Sigma) and 100 µg/mL of either PSRE or PACN and 1×10^5 bacteria. The plate was incubated 24 h at 37 °C to allow cells-bacteria direct contact. Then, cells and bacteria were detached from plate wells by a collagenase (1 mg/mL) trypsin-EDTA (0.25%) solution and collected. The number of viable cells was determined by trypan blue and Burker chamber count. Cells cultivated with fresh medium without bacteria were considered as a control.

2.5. Rat Gingival Fibroblast Cell Culture and Treatments

All experimental procedures were performed according to the Law of the Republic of Lithuanian Animal Welfare and Protection (License of the State Food and Veterinary Service for working with laboratory animals No. G2-80). The mice were maintained and handled at Lithuanian University of Health Sciences animal house in agreement with the ARRIVE guidelines. Primary gingival fibroblasts were isolated from gingiva of P5-7 rat pups. After isolation, the cells were grown in 75 cm² flasks in DMEM with high glucose and Glutamax (Thermo Fisher Scientific, Waltham, MA, USA), 10% FBS and

Pen/Strep. At 70%–90% confluence, the cells were detached by 0.025% Trypsin/EGTA and plated in 96 well plates at a density of 2×10^5 cells/well. The treatments were made 24 h after plating. All treatments were made simultaneously, without pre-incubations, and lasted 24 h. LPS was used at concentration of 2 mg/mL (1 mg/mL LPS did not induce significant increase in cell death), filtered PSRE and PACN solutions at 50 and 100 µg/mL (both preparations induced toxicity starting from 200 µg/mL).

2.6. Bone Marrow-Derived Macrophages

For bone marrow-derived macrophages (BMDM) isolation male C57BL6/J inbred mice (18–20 weeks old, Envigo, Netherlands) were used. The experimental procedures were carried out in accordance with the guidelines of the European Community (2010/63/EU), local laws and policies and were approved by the Latvian Animal Protection Ethical Committee, Food and Veterinary Service, Riga, Latvia. Mice were euthanized by decapitation, and bone marrow cells were extracted from femur bones and differentiated for 7 days in RPMI-1640 with Glutamax (Gibco,) supplemented with 10% FBS, 1% antibiotics and 10 ng/mL M-CSF (monocyte-colony stimulating factor, PeproTech, London, UK). Then cells were detached by 0.5% trypsin (Sigma Aldrich), and plated in a 12-well plate (11×10^5 cells/mL) in DMEM-high glucose medium supplemented with 10% FBS, 1% antibiotics. After 1h incubation in 37 °C incubator, cells were stimulated with PSRE and PACN at 100 µg/mL and LPS 10 ng/mL with murine IFNγ (interferon gamma, PeproTech) 100 U/mL for proinflammatory gene expression and macrophage polarization to M1 (pro-inflammatory) phenotype for 2 h and 24 h, respectively.

2.7. Human Peripheral Blood Mononuclear Cells

Human peripheral blood mononuclear cells (PBMCs) were purchased from ATCC (ATCC® PCS-800-011™, Manassas, VA, USA). The cells were cultured at 3.3×10^6 cells/mL (12 well plate) in RPMI medium supplemented with 10% FBS, 1% antibiotics. After 1 h incubation in 37 °C incubator, cells were stimulated with 1 µg/mL LPS (lipopolysaccharide, Sigma-Aldrich) in the presence of 100 µg/mL PSRE or PACN, for 6 h.

2.8. Analysis of Cell Viability by Lactate Dehydrogenase Release, Alamarblue and MTT Assay

PBMCs' viability was assessed by measuring lactate dehydrogenase (LDH) release in cell culture media. LDH activity was measured using a method based on the reduction of a tetrazolium salt (yellow) to formazan (red) [22]. The absorbance of kinetic parameters was determined spectrophotometrically at 503 nm on Hidex Sense microplate reader. The reaction mixture contained 30 mM lactate, 150 µM NAD+ (nicotinamide adenine dinucleotide), 0.4 mM 2-(4-iodophenyl)3-(4-nitrophenyl)-5-phenyltetrazolium chloride (INT) and 3.25 mM N-methylphenazonium methyl sulphate (PMS) in 100 mM Tris buffer solution (pH 8.0). In addition, PBMCs viability after 24 h incubation with different concentrations of PSRE and PACN was determined with alamarBlue®, (Bio-Rad Laboratories, Hercules, CA, USA) following the manufacturer's instructions. Briefly, the ready-to-use solution was added to each well in a 1:10 ratio and incubated for 2 h in the dark at 37 °C; then, fluorescence (Ex 544 nm/Em 590 nm) and optical density (570 and 600 nm) using Hidex Sense microplate reader.

BMDM viability after 24 incubation with different concentrations of PSRE and PACN was determined using MTT assay. After incubation, BMDM were incubated with MTT (TCI Europe) solution (1 mg/mL) for 1 h, the formazan crystals formed during incubation were dissolved in isopropanol, and optical density at 570 nm corresponding to the amount of viable cells was measured in a Hidex Sense microplate reader.

2.9. Necrosis Evaluation by Double Nuclear Staining

The level of necrotic cell death was assessed by double nuclear fluorescent staining with Hoechst33342 (10 mg/mL) and propidium iodide (PI, 5 mg/mL), 5 min at 37 °C. PI-positive nuclei indicating lost nuclear membrane integrity were considered necrotic. Cells were visualized under fluorescent microscope OLYMPUS IX71S1F-3 (Olympus Corporation, Tokyo, Japan), counted in fluorescent micrographs and expressed as the percentage of total cell number per image. The data are presented as averages ± standard deviation. LD50 was calculated by SigmaPlot v.13 (Systat Software Inc, London, UK) using the equation proposed by a dynamic curve fitting tool.

2.10. Apoptosis Evaluation by Annexin V staining

The viable cells were analyzed on a BD FACS Melody™ (BD Biosciences, San Jose, CA, USA) flow cytometer using Annexin V-allophycocyanin (BioLegend, San Diego, CA, USA) staining. For analysis of BMDMs apoptosis, treated cells were stained with fluorescent annexin V antibody and, afterwards, the proportion of apoptotic (Annexin V positive) cells was evaluated.

2.11. Caspase Activity Assessment

Caspase-3 activity in cell lysates after treatments was measured by means of a Caspase 3 Assay Kit (Sigma-Aldrich) according to the manufacturer's protocol, by assessing Ac-DEVD-7-amido-4-methylcoumarin cleavage and subsequent increase in 7-amido-4-methylcoumarin (AMC) fluorescence in a fluorometric plate reader Ascent Fluoroskan (Thermo Fisher Scientific, Waltham, MA, USA; λ_{ex} = 360 nm, λ_{em} = 460 nm). The data are presented as averages ± standard deviation of AMC concentration increase rate normalized for mg of cellular protein, averages ± standard deviation.

Caspase-8 in cell lysates after treatments was measured by means of a colorimetric Caspase 8 Assay Kit (Sigma-Aldrich) according to the manufacturer's protocol, by assessing Ac-IETD-*p*-Nitroaniline cleavage and increase in *p*-Nitroaniline (pNA) concentration in a spectrophotometric plate reader Multiskan Go 1510 (Thermo Fisher Scientific, Waltham, MA, USA) reading absorbance at λ_{ex} = 405 nm. The data are presented as averages ± standard deviation of pNA concentration increase rate normalized for mg of cellular protein, averages ± standard deviation.

2.12. Detection of Secreted Inflammatory Mediators

Medium collected after treatments was assayed for cytokines tumor necrosis factor-α (TNF-α), interleukin-6 (IL-6), interleukin-8 (IL-8) and prostaglandin E2 (PGE2) production using TNF-α mouse (Millipore), IL-6 human (Sabbiotech), IL-8 rat (Abbexa) and PGE2 rat (Abbexa) kits following the manufacturer's protocols.

2.13. Bone Marrow-Derived Macrophage Polarisation to M1 Phenotype and Analysis by Flow Cytometry

BMDMs were incubated with PSRE and PACN (100 µg/mL each) and LPS + IFNγ (10 ng/mL/100 U/mL) for 24 h. The cells were washed twice with HBSS and harvested by trypsin (0.5%), then DMEM-high glucose medium with 10% FBS was added and cell suspension was centrifuged at 300× *g* for 5 min. Then cells were incubated with specific conjugated antibody mixtures (in concentration 1:100 in cell wash buffer) for 30 min on ice in the dark. The mixture contained following monoclonal antibodies purchased from BioLegend (San Diego, CA, USA): FITC-conjugated anti-mouse F4/80, phycoerythrin (PE)-conjugated anti-mouse CD86 and biotin-conjugated anti-mouse CD80. Then cells were washed and stained with streptavidin-APC-Cy7. After 30 min, cells were washed and stained for evaluation for apoptosis (see method above). After staining samples were analyzed by flow cytometry (BD FACS Melody™, BD Biosciences, San Jose, CA, USA).

2.14. mRNA Isolation and Quantitative RT-PCR Analysis

Total RNA from cells was isolated using Ambion PureLink RNA Mini Kit (catalogue No. 12183025) according to the manufacturer's protocol. The first-strand cDNA synthesis was carried out using a High Capacity cDNA Reverse Transcription Kit (Applied Biosystems™, Foster City, CA, USA) following the manufacturer's instructions. The quantitative RT-PCR analysis of gene expression was performed by mixing SYBR Green Master Mix (Applied Biosystems™), synthesized cDNA, forward and reverse primers specific for interleukin-1β (IL-1β), interleukin 10 (IL-10), inducible nitric oxide synthase (iNOS), TNF-α, cyclooxygenase 2 (COX-2) and running the reactions on a Mic Real-Time PCR instrument. The relative expression levels for each gene were calculated with the ΔΔCt method and normalized to the expression of glucose-6-phosphate isomerase gene.

2.15. Statistical Analysis

The quantitative results are presented as mean ± standard deviation (SD) of 3–7 replicates. The data were processed using Microsoft Office Excel 2010 (Microsoft, Redmond, WA, USA) and SPSS 20 (IBM, Armonk, NY, USA) software. For antibacterial activity testing and bacterial-fibroblast co-culture experiments, the statistical data analysis was performed by applying the ANOVA with a Tukey HSD post hoc test. For experiments on rat gingival fibroblasts, ANOVA with Dunn's test was used and data analyzed by SigmaPlot v.13 (Systat Software Inc., London, UK). In all cases, differences were considered statistically significant when $p < 0.05$.

3. Results

3.1. Antibacterial Activity of Proanthocyanidins from Pelargonium sidoides Root Extract

For antibacterial efficiency evaluation, bacterial strains *S. aureus*, *S. epidermidis*, *A. actinomycetemcomitans* and *E. coli* were subjected to PSRE and PACN treatments were used at the concentration ranging from 10 to 100 µg/mL. Antibacterial activity results are summarized in Figure 1.

Both PSRE and PACN significantly reduced bacterial metabolic activity in comparison to the untreated control, starting from concentrations of 50–70 µg/mL. However, some differences were noticed between the tested strains. In the case of *S. aureus*, PSRE was more effective than PACN (Figure 1a). Fifty µg/mL of PSRE was enough to significantly decreased metabolic activity of this strain, whereas PACN had a similar result at 80 µg/mL ($p < 0.05$ vs. control, indicated by the *). For *A. actinomycetemcomitans*, the results were opposite (Figure 1d); PACN significantly decreased metabolic activity at 50 µg/mL, but it required 80 µg/mL PSRE to achieve this level of activity. The metabolism of the clinical isolate *S. epidermidis* (Figure 1b) was significantly decreased by both PSRE and PACN applied at a 70 µg/mL concentration.

Interestingly, the non-pathogen *E. coli* demonstrated the highest resistance to the treatment (Figure 1c) when the 0–80 µg/mL window was considered. After the 80 µg/mL PSRE treatment, metabolic activity of *E. coli* decreased by 26% compared with untreated control, whereas metabolic activity of *S. aureus*, *S. epidermidis* and *A. actinomycetemcomitans* was reduced by 75%, 97% and 57%, accordingly. In the presence of 80 µg/mL PACN, the loss of metabolic activity of these four strains listed in the same order was 47%, 74%, 96% and 99%. Moreover, even after addition of 100 µg/mL PACN to the growth medium, *E. coli* still preserved nearly half of the control activity level, but in the case of *A. actinomycetemcomitans*, the twice less amount of this preparation almost completely blocked bacterial growth. Summarizing, the results of the antibacterial evaluation indicate stronger toxicity of PSRE and PACN to *S. aureus*, *S. epidermidis* and *A. actinomycetemcomitans* than to non-pathogenic *E. coli* strain when the extracts were used within the 80 µg/mL range. Conversely, at higher 90 and 100 µg/mL concentrations a similar broad range effect was observed for all the tested strains as all results of both PSRE and PACN were significantly different in comparison with untreated controls ($p < 0.05$, indicated by the *).

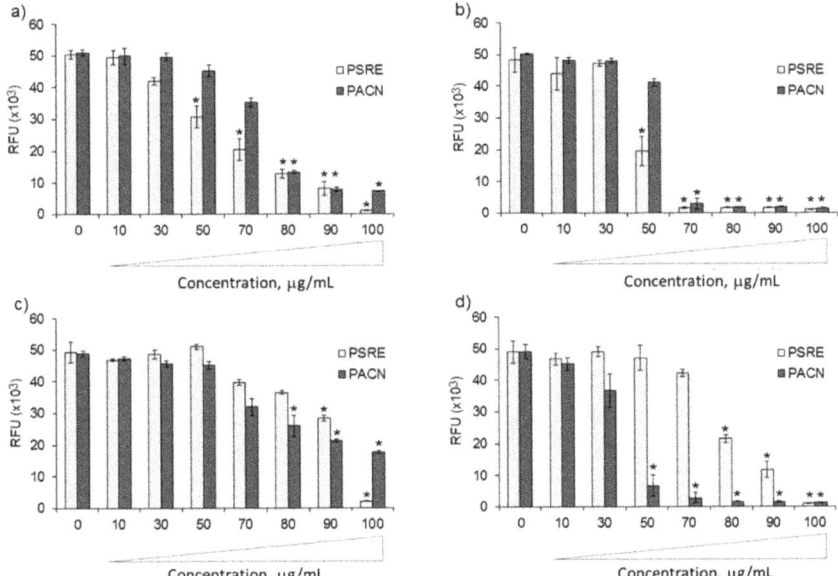

Figure 1. Antibacterial activity of *Pelargonium sidoides* root extract (PSRE) and proanthocyanidins from PSRE (PACN) towards *Staphylococcus aureus* (**a**), *S. epidermidis* (**b**), *Escherichia coli* (**c**) and *Aggregatibacter actinomycetemcomitans* (**d**). RFU—relative fluorescence units. Bars represent means and standard deviations of six experimental replicates. * = $p < 0.05$ vs. untreated control.

3.2. The Effect of Proanthocyanidins from Pelargonium sidoides Root Extract on Gingival Fibroblast Viability under Conditions of Bacterial Infection

3.2.1. *Pelargonium sidoides* Root Extract and Proanthocyanidins Preserve Gingival Fibroblasts in the Presence of Bacteria

Next in the study, we investigated whether antibacterial properties of PSRE and PACN are efficient in protecting human gingival fibroblasts during bacterial infection. For this purpose, two microenvironments were simulated: oral, by growing together gingival fibroblast cells and bacteria *A. actinomycetemcomitans*, and mucosal, by co-culturing gingival fibroblasts and *S. aureus*. Results obtained by the co-culture "race for the surface" simulation are reported in Figure 2.

Both the presence of PSRE and PACN at 100 µg/mL were effective in protecting cells from bacterial infection; the number of viable cells counted after 24 h of direct contact with bacteria was comparable with the control consisting of cells cultivated in fresh medium without bacterial presence. Conversely, when bacteria were cultivated in the same wells of cells but in the absence of PSRE or PACN (no treatment), they were able to fully colonize the well. In this scenario, no viable cells were detected for both applied models. The results indicate that the presence of either of the substances was effective in preserving gingival fibroblast cell viability by lowering bacteria proliferation.

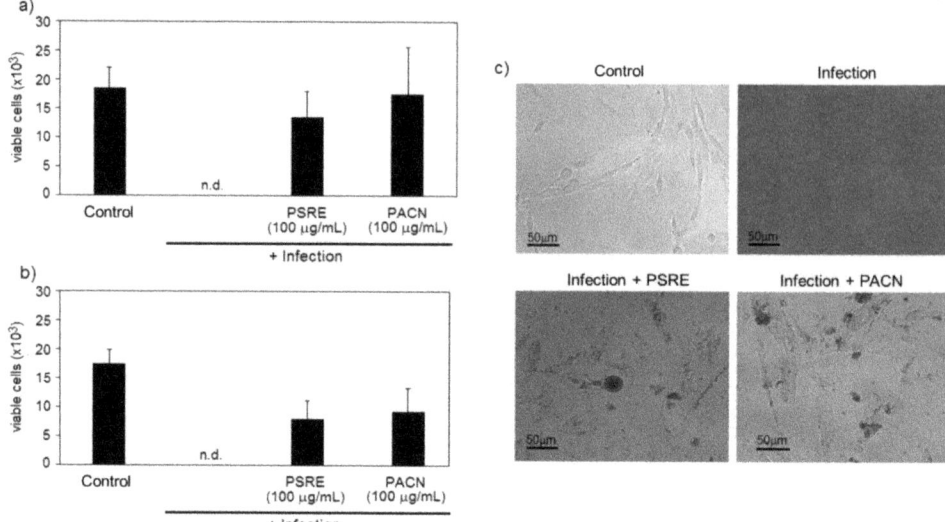

Figure 2. The effect of *Pelargonium sidoides* root extract (PSRE) and proanthocyanidins from PSRE (PACN) on human gingival fibroblast viability in co-culture "race for the surface" assay. Human gingival fibroblasts were infected with *A. actinomycetemcomitans* (**a**) or *S. aureus* (**b**); bars represent means and standard deviations of six experimental repeats. "Control" represents not infected cells, and "n.d." means there were no detectable cells in the samples. In (**c**), there are representative images of human gingival fibroblasts with *A. actinomycetemcomitans* after 24 h of infection.

3.2.2. *Pelargonium sidoides* Root Extract and Proanthocyanidins Protect Gingival Fibroblasts from Necrotic Cell Death Induced by Bacterial Lipopolysaccharide

The protective effect of PSRE and PACN under conditions of bacterial infection might be mediated not only by suppression of bacterial growth, but also by increasing the resistance of the cells to bacterial metabolites. Therefore, we examined how PSRE and PACN affect the viability of primary murine gingival fibroblasts in the presence of bacterial LPS. To select the concentrations of PSRE and PACN that has no harmful effect for the cells, the concentration-dependent toxicity was defined by double nuclear staining with propidium iodide and Hoechst33342.

The level of necrotic cells with propidium iodide-positive nuclei significantly increased after 24 h treatment with 200 μg/mL and higher concentration of both PSRE and PACN (Figure S1). PSRE demonstrated significantly higher toxicity compared to PACN in the concentration range between 200 and 350 μg/mL, and this was reflected by established LD50 for the preparations: 209 μg/mL for PSRE and 288 μg/mL for PACN. In the concentration range from 400 to 550 μg/mL, there were no further difference between the effect of both preparations and nearly all cells in the culture were found necrotic. Based on these data, there were two concentrations of PSRE and PACN selected for antiinflammatory effect study: 50 and 100 μg/mL. Both solutions were not toxic to gingival fibroblasts when applied for 24 h at these concentrations.

After treatment with 2 μg/mL LPS, the amount of necrotic cells with propidium iodide-positive nuclei in fibroblast cell culture increased from 2.7% ± 2.2% in control to 31.7% ± 11.9%, reflecting a statistically significant loss in cell viability (Figure 3). However, the treatments with 50 and 100 μg/mL PSRE and PACN prevented cell viability loss induced by LPS. The data indicate that both PSRE and PACN could protect gingival fibroblasts from bacterial LPS-induced necrosis.

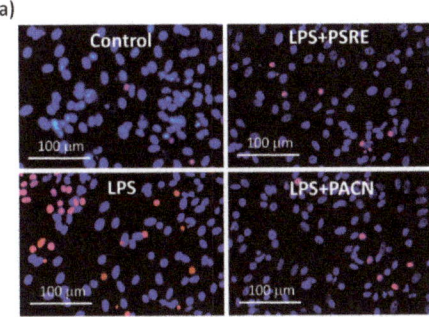 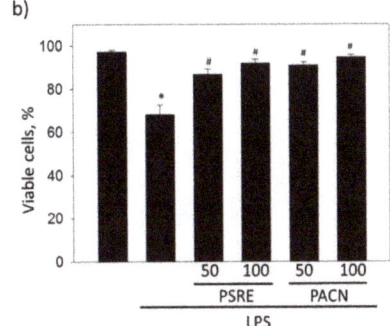

Figure 3. The effect of *Pelargonium sidoides* root extract (PSRE) and proanthocyanidins from PSRE (PACN) on the viability of gingival fibroblasts affected by bacterial lipopolysaccharide (LPS). (**a**) Representative fluorescent images after cell treatment with LPS and 100 µg/mL PSRE or PACN and nuclear viability staining; propidium iodide-positive necrotic nuclei are red, all nuclei are stained blue with Hoechst33342. (**b**) Quantitative viability results. Fifty and 100 represent the concentrations (µg/mL). The data are presented as means plus standard deviation of five experiments. *—significant difference compared to the untreated control, and #—significant difference compared to the LPS only treatment, $p < 0.05$.

3.2.3. *Pelargonium sidoides* Root Extract and Proanthocyanidin Fraction Prevent Caspase Activity Induced by Bacterial Lipopolysaccharide

Next to necrosis, bacterial toxicity might initiate apoptosis that also contributes to the loss of gingival tissue. Cysteine aspartic proteases (caspases) are key mediator enzymes in apoptosis [23]. There are two main groups of caspases according to their place in the apoptotic event cascade: initiator caspases acting as apoptotic triggers and effector caspases that are amplified by triggers and execute proteolysis leading to the characteristic biochemical and morphological changes in the apoptotic cell. To determine apoptosis-preventing capacity of PSRE and PACN, we assessed the level of active initiator caspase-8 and effector caspase-3 in LPS-treated fibroblast cells.

A 24 h LPS treatment induced elevation in caspase-8 substrate cleavage activity; it increased from 0.007 ± 0.001 nmol/min/mg in control samples to 0.047 ± 0.013 nmol/min/mg (Figure 4a). PSRE at a 50 µg/mL concentration did not significantly affect LPS-induced caspase-8 activity. However, treatments with 100 µg/mL PSRE, 50 µg/mL PACN and 100 µg/mL PACN significantly prevented caspase-8 activation by LPS by 2.2, 2.0 and 5.9 times, respectively. Treatments with 100 µg/mL PSRE and PACN without LPS had no significant effect on the activity of the caspase.

After treatment with LPS, effector caspase-3 substrate cleavage rate increased from 0.012 ± 0.01 to 0.189 ± 0.06 nmol/min/mg (Figure 4b). Both PSRE and PACN at all tested concentrations significantly reduced the effect of LPS on caspase-3 activity. When LPS was applied together with 50 µg/mL PSRE, caspase-3 activity was nearly two times lower than in LPS only-treated samples. 100 µg/mL PSRE decreased the effect of LPS on caspase-3 activity 4.7 times. Fifty and 100 µg/mL PACN lowered LPS-induced caspase-3 activity 3 and 8.8 times, respectively. There was no significant effect on caspase-3 substrate cleavage rate observed after treatment with 100 µg/mL PSRE or PACN alone, without LPS.

Overall, caspase activity evaluation indicates that both PSRE and PACN could suppress apoptotic protease activity evoked by bacterial LPS. Both preparations have a stronger effect in decreasing the executing caspase-3 activity compared with the effect on trigger caspase-8. However, PACN was more efficient in suppressing caspase-8 activity than PSRE, thus, PACN is a more powerful suppressor of apoptosis at the early stages. None of the substances was toxic to gingival fibroblasts when applied for 24 h at these concentrations.

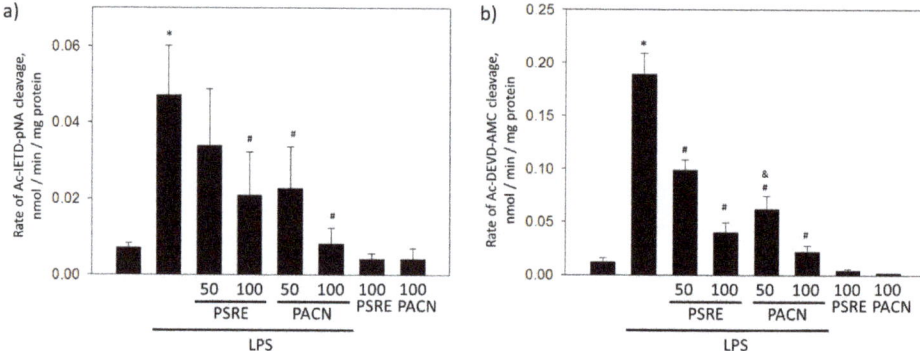

Figure 4. The effect of *Pelargonium sidoides* root extract (PSRE) and proanthocyanidins from PSRE (PACN) on LPS-induced caspase-8 (**a**) and caspase-3 (**b**) activation in gingival fibroblasts. Fifty and 100 represent the concentrations expressed in µg/mL. The data are presented as means with standard deviation of seven experimental repeats. *—significant difference compared to untreated control, #—significant difference compared to LPS only treatment and &—significant difference compared to LPS plus 50 µg/mL PSRE treatment, $p < 0.05$.

3.3. The Effect of Proanthocyanidins from Pelargonium sidoides Root Extract on Inflammatory Responses to Bacterial Lipopolysaccharide

3.3.1. The effect of *Pelargonium sidoides* Root Extract and Proanthocyanidin Fraction on Lipopolysaccharide-Induced Secretion of Inflammatory Mediators

Infection-induced inflammation is the main responsible for gingival and dental tissue loss in the pathogenesis of periodontal disease. Thus, for successful treatment of the disease it is important to defeat both infection and inflammation. Next in the study, we examined antiinflammatory properties of PSRE and PACN on LPS-induced release of inflammatory mediators from gingival fibroblasts and blood leukocytes.

Increased IL-8 production by gingival fibroblasts is responsible for attraction of neutrophils to inflamed regions and rapid tissue loss during periodontitis [24,25]. Evaluation of IL-8 amounts secreted in the medium by cultured gingival fibroblasts revealed that after 24 h with LPS the amount of the cytokine increased from nearly zero to 1022 ± 75 ng/mL (Figure 5a). In the presence of 50 µg/mL PSRE, the level of IL-8 after same LPS stimulation was only 344 ± 49 ng/mL, i.e., three times lower than without the extract. Increasing PSRE concentration to 100 µg/mL further suppressed IL-8 release to 201 ± 33 ng/mL (five times less than after LPS-only treatment). A similar suppression level was achieved by 50 µg/mL PACN, and in the presence of 100 µg/mL PACN, the level of IL-8 after LPS stimulation had further dropped to 32 ± 12 ng/mL, making the level 16 times lower than after treatment with LPS alone.

The level of PGE2, a mediator of cyclooxygenase-2 inflammatory pathway, was found to be dramatically increased in the cell culture medium after LPS treatment (Figure 5b). In control samples, the average amount of PGE2 was 5 ± 2 ng/mL, but after 24 h with LPS, it had climbed up to 2372 ± 194 ng/mL. In the presence of both 50 and 100 µg/mL PSRE, the levels of PGE2 after LPS treatment were 637 ± 58 ng/mL and 613 ± 133 ng/mL, respectively, i.e., nearly four times lower compared with the level without the extract. Treatments with 50 and 100 µg/mL PACN were even more efficient, further decreasing PGE2 level in the medium to 174 ± 41 ng/mL and 72 ± 16 ng/mL, or 14 and 33 times compared with LPS only treatment, respectively. Thus, the effects of PACN on LPS-stimulated PGE2 release were significantly stronger than those of PSRE.

Bacterial invasion also cause an infiltration of leukocytes that mediate inflammation and disturb osteoblast-osteoclast balance via release of IL-6 [23]. Thus, we investigated how PSRE and PACN affect the release of IL-6 from PBMCs. One hundred µg/mL of PSRE and PACN significantly decreased LPS-induced secretion of IL-6 from PBMCs to 67% and 18% of the level caused by LPS stimulation, respectively (Figure 5c). Note that neither PSRE nor PACN were toxic to the cells at the concentrations applied as revealed by metabolic viability analysis (Figure S2).

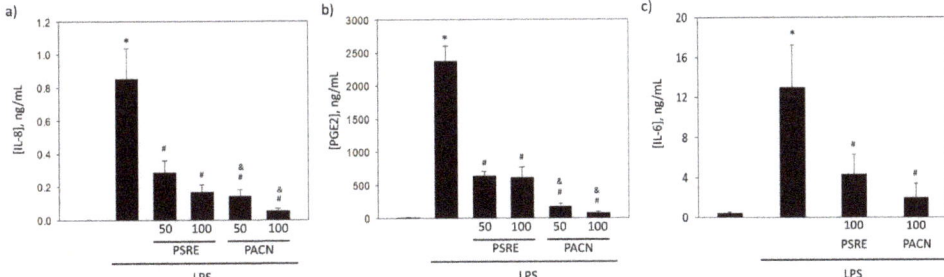

Figure 5. The effect of *Pelargonium sidoides* root extract (PSRE) and proanthocyanidins from PSRE (PACN) on (**a**) interleukin-8 (IL-8) and (**b**) prostaglandin E2 (PGE2) secretion from gingival fibroblasts, and (**c**) interleukin-6 (IL-6) secretion from peripheral blood mononuclear cells after LPS treatment. Fifty and 100 represent the concentrations (µg/mL). The data are presented as means and standard deviations of seven experiments. *—significant difference compared to untreated control, #—significant difference compared to LPS only treatment and &—significant difference compared to LPS plus a 50 µg/mL PSRE treatment, $p < 0.05$.

The data about inflammatory mediator secretion indicate that both PSRE and PACN efficiently suppress LPS-induced IL-8 and PGE2 release from gingival fibroblasts and IL-6 release from mononuclear leukocytes. PACN had slightly stronger IL-8 and IL-6 release suppressing activity, and significantly stronger PGE2 release suppressing activity than PSRE.

3.3.2. The Effect of *Pelargonium sidoides* Root Extract and Proanthocyanidin Fraction on Lipopolysaccharide-Induced Expression of Inflammation-Related Genes

The release of inflammatory factors is the first step of innate immune response to pathogens. The next step leading to prolonged and enhanced inflammatory reaction is induction of inflammatory genes to produce new mediators. If uncontrolled at this stage, acute inflammation may become chronic and contribute to tissue loss in periodontitis. Activated macrophages and leukocytes are the main source of interleukin-1β (IL-1β) and TNF-α, the acute phase pyrogenic cytokines involved in most of the processes that maintain inflammation [26]. Bacterial infection also triggers inducible NO synthases (iNOS) to produce reactive nitrogen species stress on pathogens [27]. Therefore, we have examined the capacity of PSRE and PACN to modulate expression of inflammatory genes IL-1β, TNF-α and iNOS in primary murine bone marrow-derived macrophages and human mononuclear leukocytes under treatment of LPS. Stimulation of macrophages in the presence of interferon-γ (IFN-γ) acting as enhancer of LPS-induced gene expression [28] induced an increase in transcription of all the three genes investigated (Figure 6a–c).

Both preparations at a dose of 100 µg/mL significantly suppressed the mRNA transcription of IL-1β and iNOS (Figure 6a,b). The level of the IL-1β mRNA decreased by 78% of the initial level with LPS after treatment with PSRE, and by 89%—after treatment with PACN. For iNOS, the decrease in mRNA level after PSRE and PACN treatment was 53% and 64%, respectively. However, the incubation with both substances did not affect LPS plus IFN-γ-induced TNF-α gene expression (Figure 6c). 6 h treatment with LPS caused significant increase in cyclooxygenase-2 (COX-2), TNF-α and IL-1β gene transcription in human PBMCs (Figure 6d–f). PSRE and PACN at a concentration of 100 µg/mL significantly suppressed mRNA transcription of COX-2 and IL-1β. When LPS was together with PSRE, COX-2 and IL-1β mRNA levels dropped by 50%, 73% and 56%, respectively. For PACN, mRNA synthesis for these cytokines was suppressed by 63%, 89% and 76%. Similarly to BMDMs case, neither PSRE, nor PACN significantly affected TNF-α gene expression. Both PSRE and PACN at a concentration of 100 μg/mL were not toxic for PBMCs and BMDMs as revealed by metabolic activity and apoptosis evaluation (Supplementary Figures S2 and S3).

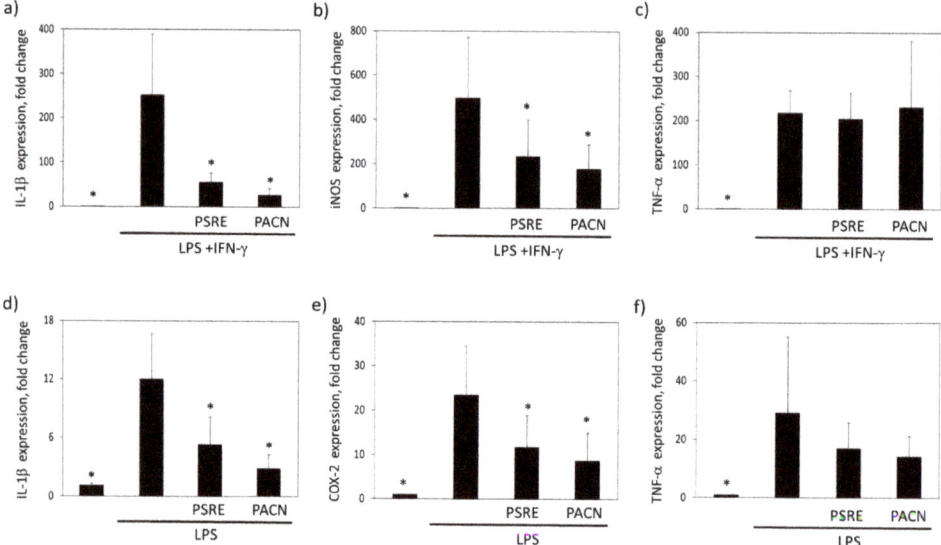

Figure 6. The effect of *Pelargonium sidoides* root extract (PSRE) and proanthocyanidins from PSRE (PACN) on proinflammatory gene expression in bone marrow-derived macrophages (**a–c**) and peripheral blood mononuclear cells (**d–f**) after LPS or LPS and IFN- stimulation. (**a,d**) IL-1β (**a,b**) iNOS, (**c,f**) TNF- and (**e**) COX-2. The data are expressed as a fold change of glucose-6-phosphate isomerase gene transcription and presented as mean ± SD of three independent measurements. *—significantly different from the LPS-treated samples (ANOVA followed by a Tukey's multiple comparison test, $p < 0.05$).

The gene expression analysis indicate that both preparations acted as inflammatory signal suppressors preventing expression of pro-inflammatory cytokine IL-1β and prostaglandin producing enzyme COX-2 genes, as well as decreasing synthesis of iNOS and protecting tissues from the damage of reactive nitrogen species. However, neither PSRE nor PACN significantly influenced TNF-α gene expression.

3.3.3. The Effect of *Pelargonium sidoides* Root Extract and Proanthocyanidin Fraction on Lipopolysaccharide-Induced Macrophage Conversion to M1 Phenotype

Activated macrophages can be polarized into a proinflammatory M1 phenotype and alternative anti-inflammatory M2 phenotype [29]. Increase in the M1/M2 macrophage ratio can lead from an antibacterial defense to the development of periodontitis and positively correlates with the severity of the disease [30]. Next in the study, we tested how PSRE and PACN affect LPS and IFN-γ-stimulated macrophage polarization to proinflammatory M1 phenotype characterized by the presentation of surface markers CD80 and CD86 [31,32].

Flow cytometry analysis revealed that in response to LPS and IFN-γ, the amount of M1-polarised macrophages increased 9.3 times compared to the untreated control (Figure 7). Both PSRE and PACN at a concentration of 100 μg/mL were effective in reducing the level of CD80 and CD86-positive cells. The population of cells with the exposed markers after treatment with PSRE was by 58% lower, and after treatment with PACN by 71% lower than after LPS and IFN-γ stimulation without the treatments. The results indicate that both substances were potent in preventing macrophage conversion to proinflammatory M1 phenotype under exposure to LPS and IFN-γ treatment.

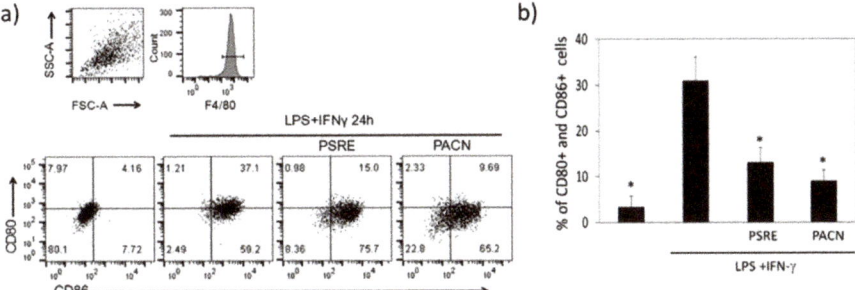

Figure 7. Expression of proinflammatory cell surface markers CD80 and CD86 analyzed by flow cytometry 24 h after treating LPS + IFNγ-activated BMDMs with PSRE and PACN. (**a**) Characteristic mouse macrophage marker F4/80-positive cells were gated for double CD80 and CD86 analysis as a measure of M1 macrophage phenotype (top right small quadrant). Representative plots of a total of three independent experiments in three replicates are presented in the bottom. (**b**) Mean ± SD of three independent measurements in three parallels. Differences between the measurements were tested using a one-way ANOVA followed by a Tukey's multiple comparison test. *—significantly different from the LPS and IFN-γ treatment ($p < 0.05$).

4. Discussion

Increasing antibiotic resistance makes the search for alternative antimicrobial compounds of a crucial importance for global health [33]. Failure to defeat fast adapting pathogens without significant damage to host tissues is a key challenge in management of chronic infectious-inflammatory disease including periodontitis [34]. Progressive bacteria-driven inflammatory response causes continuous damage on periodontal cells making them more sensitive to harmful effects of antibiotics and antimicrobial chemicals [3,35]. The damage is further exacerbated by the treatment-caused loss of beneficial commensal bacteria [36]. This suggests reconsidering the possibilities of alternative treatment strategies including use of specific pathogen-targeting bacterial strains [37] and plant-derived antibacterials, because such strategies are characterized by lower or no side effects and resistance development risk, as well as complex antiinflammatory and tissue renewal stimulating properties. This study explored antibacterial and antiinflammatory properties of PSRE that is known as potent infection-defeating preparation and PSRE-derived PACN possessing stronger antioxidant and antibacterial properties compared to PSRE [17,19].

Both substances were effective in reducing metabolic activity of the selected strains suggesting a broad range of antibacterial properties. This is in line with previous evidence about various extracts prepared from *P. sidoides* roots. A commercial aqueous-ethanolic extract from *P. sidoides* EPs® 7630 (Umckaloabo®) is reported to inhibit growth of *Streptococcus pyogenes*, *Proteus mirabilis*, *Staphylococcus aureus*, *Escherichia coli*, *Streptococcus pneumoniae*, *Haemophilus influenza*, *Staphylococcus epidermidis* and some other gram-negative and gram-positive bacterial strains (summarized in [38]). Aqueous-acetone PSRE was efficient in decreasing growth of antibiotic-resistant *S. aureus* strains [39]. The present study for the first time demonstrated the growth-suppressing efficiency of PSRE and PACN on *Aggregatibacter actinomycetemcomitans*, one of the most important gram-negative anaerobic periodontal pathogens [40]. Similarly as in the previously demonstrated case of *P. gingivalis* [19], PACN demonstrated significantly higher toxicity on *A. actinomycetemcomitans*, compared to the effect of PSRE. Fifty µg/mL PACN reduced metabolic activity of *A. actinomycetemcomitans* nearly 10 times more if compared to the untreated control value (Figure 1d). The same concentration had no significant toxicity on other investigated strains. The minimal amount of PACN causing a significant effect on metabolic activity of *E. coli* and *S. aureus* was 80 µg/mL, and for *S. epidermidis* the significant toxicity started from 70 µg/mL PACN. The results indicate that there might be a specific interaction of proanthocyanidins from PSRE with the main pathogenic strains (*P. gingivalis* and *A. actinomycetemcomitans*) responsible for the development of periodontitis. Strain-specific activity of proanthocyanidins was already noticed by other authors. Lacombe and Wu have reviewed the selective pathogen-suppressing and beneficial strain-promoting activity of proanthocyanidins derived from various berries [41]. However, despite many publications reporting a selective activity of natural extracts towards pathogen and non-pathogen strains, it is still not completely clear how this selection occurs [42]. It was shown that cranberry-derived proanthocyanidins are able to interfere with a N-acylhomoserine lactone-mediated quorum sensing of *Pseudomonas aeruginosa* [43]. Moreover, proanthocyanidins have also been shown to compromise adhesion to host cells by mimicking cell surface signaling [44]. Some authors have proposed the hypothesis that proanthocyanidins might increase bacterial membrane permeability and cause indirect metabolism decrease due to ATP and other intracellular metabolite loss [42,45]. A recent study shows that proanthocyanidins can potentiate antibiotics by acting via bacterial multidrug efflux pumps [46]. Thus, the disturbance in transmembrane transport indeed might be the cause of bacteriotoxicity. However, more studies definitely are required to clarify the mechanism of action of proanthocyanidins against pathogenic bacterial strains.

On the other hand, PSRE was more efficient than PACN in suppressing both of *Staphylococcus* strains that were investigated in this study suggesting that other than proanthocyanidin fraction compounds were acting against these bacteria. Most likely, the distinct antibacterial activity of PSRE can be ascribed to other phenolic compounds such as coumarins, phenolic acids, flavonols and flavan-3-ols [16].

Bacterial infection simulation in the co-culture "race for the surface" assay revealed that addition of 100 µg/mL of either PSRE or PACN in the medium was effective in preserving viability of human gingival fibroblasts in the presence of both *S. aureus* and *A. actinomycetemcomitans* (Figure 2). Similarly, B-type linked proanthocyanidin-coated surfaces are shown to inhibit bacterial spreading and promote survival of mammalian cells [47]. The mechanism proposed to explain the activity is bacterial attachment and biofilm formation prevention by prodelphinidin-rich proanthocyanidins. In our experimental model, a similar efficiency was achieved by PSRE and PACN solutions, indicating that interaction of soluble compounds with the walls of bacteria also could mediate bacterial adhesion and mammalian cell protection. Accordingly, these results are very promising support to the use of natural extracts as an effective alternative antibacterial compound able to preserve the naïve tissue.

Investigation of gingival tissue protecting properties of PSRE and PACN in the bacterial LPS-mediated inflammation model revealed that both preparations efficiently prevent necrosis and apoptosis of fibroblast cells. Both substances were more efficient in decreasing the executing caspase-3 activity compared with the effect on apoptosis triggering caspase-8. However, PSRE was less efficient in suppressing caspase-8 activity than PACN, indicating that the latter had both upstream and downstream targets in the apoptotic cascade. The antiapoptotic activity of proanthocyanidins from grape seeds including decrease in executing caspases-3 and 9 was reported in a rotenone-induced neurotoxicity model of SH-SY5Y cells [48]. However, exposure of human colorectal carcinoma cells HCT-116 to proanthocyanidins from the same source significantly upregulated mRNAs encoding caspase-2, caspase-3 and caspase-9 [49]. Another study reports apoptosis induction in lung cancer cells NCI-H460 via stimulation of caspase-3 and mitochondrial cytochrome c release by gallic acid, one of the important constituents of PSRE [50]. Such controversial data suggest that the effect of PSRE and proanthocyanidins on apoptotic signaling pathways is cell type-dependent and they might have opposite effects in cancerous and non-cancerous cells as well as in different toxicity models.

Evaluation of pro-inflammatory cytokine secretion and gene expression revealed that PSRE and PACN suppress at least three different inflammatory processes: cytokine secretion (IL-8 from gingival fibroblasts and IL-6 from bone marrow-derived macrophages), inflammatory gene expression (IL-1β, iNOS and COX-2) and macrophage conversion to pro-inflammatory M1 phenotype related to the tissue loss in periodontitis. Downregulation of COX-2 coding mRNA in mononuclear leukocytes and PGE2 release from gingival fibroblasts indicate suppression of the prostaglandin inflammatory pathway. PGE2 is the most prominent in the pathogenesis of periodontitis among prostaglandins [51,52]. PGE2 is involved in the stimulation of inflammatory mediators and MMPs, as well as osteoclast formation via receptor activator of nuclear factor-κB ligand (RANKL) [52,53]. IL-6 and IL-1β also mediate bone resorption via osteoclasts activation [54], and increase in iNOS leads to reactive nitrogen species-mediated apoptosis of gingival fibroblasts [55]. By suppressing these inflammatory pathways, PSRE and PACN are expected to significantly improve condition and survival of periodontal tissues. Similar antiinflammatory activity of PSRE together with *Coptis chinensis* root extract was recently shown in LPS-stimulated RAW 264.7 cells [56]. The extract combination significantly decreased the levels of iNOS, PGE2, TNF-α, IL-1β and IL-6 in RAW 264.7 macrophages, and the results were also confirmed in vivo in a paw oedema rat model. Although the study reported lower levels of TNF-α secretion from LPS-stimulated RAW 264.7 cells, in our study, we did not observe significant changes on TNF-α gene expression in both LPS-stimulated leukocytes and LPS/IFN-γ-stimulated macrophages after PSRE and PACN treatment. Proinflammatory cytokine TNF-α plays a critical role not only in inflammatory cell migration, but also in both innate and adaptive immune responses, by up-regulating antigen presentation and the bactericidal activity of phagocytes [57,58]. In periodontitis, TNF-α is one of the key signals initiating several signaling pathways leading to chemotaxis of other inflammatory cells, tissue destruction and osteoclast formation [59,60]. The fact that PSRE and PACN had no effect on TNF-α expression level while suppressing several other related genes indicate the targets of the substances are located either downstream of the TNF-α signal or in the TNF-a excluding pathway.

Although antiinflammatory properties of PACN and PSRE revealed in the study were of comparative levels, PACN had stronger efficiency in suppressing caspases and preventing mediator release. Stronger anti-inflammatory activity of PACN might be due to greater amounts of prodelphinidins. These compounds possess higher antioxidant capacity and share certain important structural peculiarities, namely hydroxyl groups in B ring (especially in C4' position and catechol group), hydroxyl groups in the A ring at the C5 and C7 positions [61].

5. Conclusions

In conclusion, both PSRE and PACN revealed antibacterial and antiinflammatory efficiency in periodontitis mimicking conditions. However, the combination of strong pathogen-selective antibacterial, antiinflammatory and gingival tissue protecting properties of PACN suggests this preparation as a potential candidate for treatment and prevention of periodontal disease.

Supplementary Materials: The following are available online at http://www.mdpi.com/2072-6643/11/11/2829/s1, Figure S1: The concentration-dependent toxicity of *Pelargonium sidoides* root extract (PSRE) and proanthocyanidins from PSRE (PACN) for rat gingival fibroblasts, Figure S2: Effects of *Pelargonium sidoides* root extract (PSRE) and proanthocyanidins from PSRE (PACN) on human peripheral blood mononuclear cell viability, Figure S3: The effect of Pelargonium sidoides DC root extract (PSRE) and proanthocyanidins from PSRE (PACN) on Detection of apoptosis by staining bone-marrow derived macrophages (BMDM).

Author Contributions: Conceptualization, M.D., A.J., L.R. (Lia Rimondini), and N.S.; methodology, M.D., A.J., L.R. (Lia Rimondini), A.C., I.S., M.M.-K., E.M., L.R. (Lina Raudone); investigation, I.S., A.C., M.M.-K., G.L., E.M., R.B. (Rasa Bernotiene), E.V., L.R. (Lina Raudone), R.B. (Rasa Baniene), A.S.; data curation, I.S., A.C., M.M.-K., E.M., G.L., A.J.; writing—original draft preparation, A.J., M.D., A.C.; writing—review and editing, All authors; supervision, M.D., A.J., L.R. (Lia Rimondini), N.S.; funding acquisition, N.S., M.D., L.R. (Lia Rimondini).

Funding: This research is a part of the project PELARGODONT ("Engineering and functionalization of delivery system with *Pelargonium sidoides* biologically active substance on inflamed periodontal surface area") funded by a grant (No. S-M-ERA.NET-17-2) from the Research Council of Lithuania, the State Education Development Agency of Latvia, and Italian Ministry of Education, University and Research.

Conflicts of Interest: The authors declare no conflict of interest.

References

1. Loesche, W.J.; Grossman, N.S. Periodontal Disease as a Specific, albeit Chronic, Infection: Diagnosis and Treatment. *Clin. Microbiol. Rev.* **2001**, *14*, 727. [CrossRef]
2. Khan, S.A.; Kong, E.F.; Meiller, T.F.; Jabra-Rizk, M.A. Periodontal Diseases: Bug Induced, Host Promoted. *PLoS Pathog.* **2015**, *11*, e1004952. [CrossRef]
3. Soares, G.M.S.; Figueiredo, L.C.; Faveri, M.; Cortelli, S.C.; Duarte, P.M.; Feres, M. Mechanisms of action of systemic antibiotics used in periodontal treatment and mechanisms of bacterial resistance to these drugs. *J. Appl. Oral Sci.* **2012**, *20*, 295–309. [CrossRef]
4. Pareek, V.; Gupta, R.; Panwar, J. Do physico-chemical properties of silver nanoparticles decide their interaction with biological media and bactericidal action? A review. *Mater. Sci. Eng. C* **2018**, *90*, 739–749. [CrossRef]
5. Nakatsuji, T.; Chen, T.H.; Narala, S.; Chun, K.A.; Two, A.M.; Yun, T.; Shafiq, F.; Kotol, P.F.; Bouslimani, A.; Melnik, A.V.; et al. Antimicrobials from human skin commensal bacteria protect against Staphylococcus aureus and are deficient in atopic dermatitis. *Sci. Transl. Med.* **2017**, *9*. [CrossRef]
6. Avila, M.; Ojcius, D.M.; Yilmaz, O. The oral microbiota: Living with a permanent guest. *DNA Cell Biol.* **2009**, *28*, 405–411. [CrossRef]
7. Brambilla, E.; Ionescu, A.; Gagliani, M.; Cochis, A.; Arciola, C.R.; Rimondini, L. Biofilm Formation on Composite Resins for Dental Restorations: An in Situ Study on the Effect of Chlorhexidine Mouthrinses. *Int. J. Artif. Organs* **2012**, *35*, 792–799. [CrossRef]
8. Azzimonti, B.; Cochis, A.; Beyrouthy, M.; Iriti, M.; Uberti, F.; Sorrentino, R.; Landini, M.M.; Rimondini, L.; Varoni, E.M. Essential Oil from Berries of Lebanese Juniperus excelsa M. Bieb Displays Similar Antibacterial Activity to Chlorhexidine but Higher Cytocompatibility with Human Oral Primary Cells. *Molecules* **2015**, *20*, 9344–9357. [CrossRef]
9. Singh, N.; Savita, S.; Rithesh, K.; Shivanand, S. Phytotherapy: A novel approach for treating periodontal disease. *J. Pharm. Biomed. Sci. JPBMS.* **2010**, *6*, 205–210.
10. Santos-Buelga, C.; Scalbert, A. Proanthocyanidins and tannin-like compounds—Nature, occurrence, dietary intake and effects on nutrition and health. *J. Sci. Food Agric.* **2000**, *80*, 1094–1117. [CrossRef]
11. Aron, P.M.; Kennedy, J.A. Flavan-3-ols: Nature, occurrence and biological activity. *Mol. Nutr. Food Res.* **2008**, *52*, 79–104. [CrossRef]
12. Raudone, L.; Vilkickyte, G.; Pitkauskaite, L.; Raudonis, R.; Vainoriene, R.; Motiekaityte, V.; Raudone, L.; Vilkickyte, G.; Pitkauskaite, L.; Raudonis, R.; et al. Antioxidant Activities of Vaccinium vitis-idaea L. Leaves within Cultivars and Their Phenolic Compounds. *Molecules* **2019**, *24*, 844. [CrossRef]
13. Balalaie, A.; Rezvani, M.B.; Basir, M.M. Dual function of proanthocyanidins as both MMP inhibitor and crosslinker in dentin biomodification: A literature review. *Dent. Mater. J.* **2018**, *37*, 173–182. [CrossRef]
14. Shahzad, M.; Millhouse, E.; Culshaw, S.; Edwards, C.A.; Ramage, G.; Combet, E. Selected dietary (poly)phenols inhibit periodontal pathogen growth and biofilm formation. *Food Funct.* **2015**, *6*, 719–729. [CrossRef]
15. Kolodziej, H. Aqueous ethanolic extract of the roots of Pelargonium sidoides—New scientific evidence for an old anti-infective phytopharmaceutical. *Planta Med.* **2008**, *74*, 661–666. [CrossRef]
16. Kayser, O.; Kolodziej, H. Antibacterial Activity of Extracts and Constituents of *Pelargonium sidoides* and *Pelargonium reniforme*. *Planta Med.* **1997**, *63*, 508–510. [CrossRef]
17. Kolodziej, H. Antimicrobial, antiviral and immunomodulatory activity studies of pelargonium sidoides (EPs® 7630) in the context of health promotion. *Pharmaceuticals* **2011**, *4*, 1295–1314. [CrossRef]
18. Janecki, A.; Conrad, A.; Engels, I.; Frank, U.; Kolodziej, H. Evaluation of an aqueous-ethanolic extract from Pelargonium sidoides (EPs® 7630) for its activity against group A-streptococci adhesion to human HEp-2 epithelial cells. *J. Ethnopharmacol.* **2011**, *133*, 147–152. [CrossRef]
19. Savickiene, N.; Jekabsone, A.; Raudone, L.; Abdelgeliel, A.; Cochis, A.; Rimondini, L.; Makarova, E.; Grinberga, S.; Pugovics, O.; Dambrova, M.; et al. Efficacy of Proanthocyanidins from Pelargonium sidoides Root Extract in Reducing P. gingivalis Viability While Preserving Oral Commensal S. salivarius. *Materials* **2018**, *11*, 1499. [CrossRef]
20. Gristina, A.G.; Naylor, P.T.; Myrvik, Q. The Race for the Surface: Microbes, Tissue Cells, and Biomaterials. In *Molecular Mechanisms of Microbial Adhesion*; Springer: New York, NY, USA, 1989; pp. 177–211.
21. Hellström, J.; Sinkkonen, J.; Maarit Karonen, A.; Mattila, P. Isolation and Structure Elucidation of Procyanidin Oligomers from Saskatoon Berries (Amelanchier alnifolia). *J. Agric. Food Chem.* **2006**. [CrossRef]

22. Buttery, J.E.; Lim, H.H.; De Witt, G.F. The use of NADH as a standard in a modified PMS-INT colorimetric assay of lactate dehydrogenase. *Clin. Chim. Acta* **1976**, *73*, 109–115. [CrossRef]
23. Chang, H.Y.; Yang, X. Proteases for cell suicide: Functions and regulation of caspases. *Microbiol. Mol. Biol. Rev.* **2000**, *64*, 821–846. [CrossRef] [PubMed]
24. Rashmi, S.; Alka, D.; Ramakant, S. Neutrophils in health and disease: An overview. *J. Oral Maxillofac. Pathol.* **2006**, *10*, 3. [CrossRef]
25. Dongari-Bagtzoglou, A.I.; Ebersole, J.L. Increased Presence of Interleukin-6 (IL-6) and IL-8 Secreting Fibroblast Subpopulations in Adult Periodontitis. *J. Periodontol.* **1998**, *69*, 899–910. [CrossRef]
26. Arango Duque, G.; Descoteaux, A. Macrophage cytokines: Involvement in immunity and infectious diseases. *Front. Immunol.* **2014**, *5*, 491. [CrossRef]
27. Xue, Q.; Yan, Y.; Zhang, R.; Xiong, H. Regulation of iNOS on Immune Cells and Its Role in Diseases. *Int. J. Mol. Sci.* **2018**, *19*, 3805. [CrossRef]
28. Held, T.K.; Weihua, X.; Yuan, L.; Kalvakolanu, D.V.; Cross, A.S. Gamma interferon augments macrophage activation by lipopolysaccharide by two distinct mechanisms, at the signal transduction level and via an autocrine mechanism involving tumor necrosis factor alpha and interleukin-1. *Infect. Immun.* **1999**, *67*, 206–212.
29. Barrett, J.P.; Costello, D.A.; O'Sullivan, J.; Cowley, T.R.; Lynch, M.A. Bone marrow-derived macrophages from aged rats are more responsive to inflammatory stimuli. *J. Neuroinflammation* **2015**, *12*, 67. [CrossRef]
30. Zhou, L.; Bi, C.; Gao, L.; An, Y.; Chen, F.; Chen, F. Macrophage polarization in human gingival tissue in response to periodontal disease. *Oral Dis.* **2019**, *25*, 265–273. [CrossRef]
31. Orecchioni, M.; Ghosheh, Y.; Pramod, A.B.; Ley, K. Macrophage Polarization: Different Gene Signatures in M1(LPS+) vs. Classically and M2(LPS−) vs. Alternatively Activated Macrophages. *Front. Immunol.* **2019**, *10*, 1084. [CrossRef]
32. Lambert, C.; Preijers, F.W.M.B.; Yanikkaya Demirel, G.; Sack, U. Monocytes and macrophages in flow: An ESCCA initiative on advanced analyses of monocyte lineage using flow cytometry. *Cytom. Part B Clin. Cytom.* **2017**, *92*, 180–188. [CrossRef]
33. Ventola, C.L. The antibiotic resistance crisis: Part 1: Causes and threats. *Pharm. Ther.* **2015**, *40*, 277–283.
34. Shaddox, L.M.; Walker, C.B. Treating chronic periodontitis: Current status, challenges, and future directions. *Clin. Cosmet. Investig. Dent.* **2010**, *2*, 79–91. [CrossRef]
35. Seymour, R.A. Effects of medications on the periodontal tissues in health and disease. *Periodontol. 2000* **2006**, *40*, 120–129. [CrossRef]
36. Irie, K.; Novince, C.M.; Darveau, R.P. Impact of the Oral Commensal Flora on Alveolar Bone Homeostasis. *J. Dent. Res.* **2014**, *93*, 801–806. [CrossRef]
37. Patini, R.; Cattani, P.; Marchetti, S.; Isola, G.; Quaranta, G.; Gallenzi, P. Evaluation of Predation Capability of Periodontopathogens Bacteria by Bdellovibrio Bacteriovorus HD100. An in Vitro Study. *Materials* **2019**, *12*, 2008. [CrossRef]
38. Moyo, M.; Van Staden, J. Medicinal properties and conservation of Pelargonium sidoides DC. *J. Ethnopharmacol.* **2014**, *152*, 243–255. [CrossRef]
39. Kolodziej, H.; Kayser, O.; Radtke, O.A.; Kiderlen, A.F.; Koch, E. Pharmacological profile of extracts of Pelargonium sidoides and their constituents. *Phytomedicine* **2003**, *10*, 18–24. [CrossRef]
40. Benso, B. Virulence factors associated with Aggregatibacter actinomycetemcomitans and their role in promoting periodontal diseases. *Virulence* **2017**, *8*, 111–114. [CrossRef]
41. Lacombe, A.; Wu, V.C.H. The potential of berries to serve as selective inhibitors of pathogens and promoters of beneficial microorganisms. *Food Qual. Saf.* **2017**, *1*, 3–12. [CrossRef]
42. Thapa, D.; Losa, R.; Zweifel, B.; Wallace, R.J. Sensitivity of pathogenic and commensal bacteria from the human colon to essential oils. *Microbiology* **2012**, *158*, 2870–2877. [CrossRef]
43. Maisuria, V.B.; Los Santos, Y.L.; Tufenkji, N.; Déziel, E. Cranberry-derived proanthocyanidins impair virulence and inhibit quorum sensing of Pseudomonas aeruginosa. *Sci. Rep.* **2016**, *6*, 30169. [CrossRef]
44. Krachler, A.M.; Orth, K. Targeting the bacteria-host interface: Strategies in anti-adhesion therapy. *Virulence* **2013**, *4*, 284–294. [CrossRef]
45. Di Pasqua, R.; Betts, G.; Hoskins, N.; Edwards, M.; Ercolini, D.; Mauriello, G. Membrane Toxicity of Antimicrobial Compounds from Essential Oils. *J. Agric. Food Chem.* **2007**, *55*, 4863–4870. [CrossRef]

46. Maisuria, V.B.; Okshevsky, M.; Déziel, E.; Tufenkji, N. Proanthocyanidin Interferes with Intrinsic Antibiotic Resistance Mechanisms of Gram-Negative Bacteria. *Adv. Sci.* **2019**, *6*, 1802333. [CrossRef]
47. Trentin, D.S.; Silva, D.B.; Frasson, A.P.; Rzhepishevska, O.; da Silva, M.V.; Pulcini, E.D.L.; James, G.; Soares, G.V.; Tasca, T.; Ramstedt, M.; et al. Natural Green coating inhibits adhesion of clinically important bacteria. *Sci. Rep.* **2015**, *5*, 8287. [CrossRef]
48. Ma, J.; Gao, S.S.; Yang, H.J.; Wang, M.; Cheng, B.F.; Feng, Z.W.; Wang, L. Neuroprotective Effects of Proanthocyanidins, Natural Flavonoids Derived From Plants, on Rotenone-Induced Oxidative Stress and Apoptotic Cell Death in Human Neuroblastoma SH-SY5Y Cells. *Front. Neurosci.* **2018**, *12*, 369. [CrossRef]
49. Zhang, C.; Chen, W.; Zhang, X.; Zheng, Y.; Yu, F.; Liu, Y.; Wang, Y. Grape seed proanthocyanidins induce mitochondrial pathway-mediated apoptosis in human colorectal carcinoma cells. *Oncol. Lett.* **2017**, *14*, 5853–5860. [CrossRef]
50. Ji, B.C.; Hsu, W.H.; Yang, J.S.; Hsia, T.C.; Lu, C.C.; Chiang, J.H.; Yang, J.L.; Lin, C.H.; Lin, J.J.; Suen, L.J.W.; et al. Gallic Acid Induces Apoptosis via Caspase-3 and Mitochondrion-Dependent Pathways in Vitro and Suppresses Lung Xenograft Tumor Growth in Vivo. *J. Agric. Food Chem.* **2009**, *57*, 7596–7604. [CrossRef]
51. Hikiji, H.; Takato, T.; Shimizu, T.; Ishii, S. The roles of prostanoids, leukotrienes, and platelet-activating factor in bone metabolism and disease. *Prog. Lipid Res.* **2008**, *47*, 107–126. [CrossRef]
52. Noguchi, K.; Ishikawa, I. The roles of cyclooxygenase-2 and prostaglandin E_2 in periodontal disease. *Periodontol. 2000* **2007**, *43*, 85–101. [CrossRef] [PubMed]
53. Kaneko, H.; Mehrotra, M.; Alander, C.; Lerner, U.; Pilbeam, C.; Raisz, L. Effects of prostaglandin E2 and lipopolysaccharide on osteoclastogenesis in RAW 264.7 cells. *Prostaglandins Leukot. Essent. Fat. Acids* **2007**, *77*, 181–186. [CrossRef]
54. Hienz, S.A.; Paliwal, S.; Ivanovski, S. Mechanisms of Bone Resorption in Periodontitis. *J. Immunol. Res.* **2015**, *2015*, 615486. [CrossRef] [PubMed]
55. Ghosh, A.; Park, J.Y.; Fenno, C.; Kapila, Y.L. Porphyromonas gingivalis, gamma interferon, and a proapoptotic fibronectin matrix form a synergistic trio that induces c-Jun N-terminal kinase 1-mediated nitric oxide generation and cell death. *Infect. Immun.* **2008**, *76*, 5514–5523. [CrossRef] [PubMed]
56. Park, S.M.; Min, B.G.; Jung, J.Y.; Jegal, K.H.; Lee, C.W.; Kim, K.Y.; Kim, Y.W.; Choi, Y.W.; Cho, I.J.; Ku, S.K.; et al. Combination of Pelargonium sidoides and Coptis chinensis root inhibits nuclear factor kappa B-mediated inflammatory response in vitro and in vivo. *BMC Complement. Altern. Med.* **2018**, *18*. [CrossRef]
57. Dinarello, C.A. Proinflammatory Cytokines. *Chest* **2000**, *118*, 503–508. [CrossRef]
58. Garlet, G.P.; Cardoso, C.R.B.; Campanelli, A.P.; Ferreira, B.R.; Avila-Campos, M.J.; Cunha, F.Q.; Silva, J.S. The dual role of p55 tumour necrosis factor-alpha receptor in Actinobacillus actinomycetemcomitans-induced experimental periodontitis: Host protection and tissue destruction. *Clin. Exp. Immunol.* **2007**, *147*, 128–138. [CrossRef]
59. Graves, D.T.; Cochran, D. The Contribution of Interleukin-1 and Tumor Necrosis Factor to Periodontal Tissue Destruction. *J. Periodontol.* **2003**, *74*, 391–401. [CrossRef]
60. Yucel-Lindberg, T.; Båge, T. Inflammatory mediators in the pathogenesis of periodontitis. *Expert Rev. Mol. Med.* **2013**, *15*, e7. [CrossRef]
61. Ambriz-Ambriz-Pérez, D.L.; Leyva-Lopez, N.; Gutierrez-Grijalva, E.P.; Heredia, J.B. Phenolic compounds: Natural alternative in inflammation treatment. A Review. *Cogent Food Agric.* **2016**, *2*. [CrossRef]

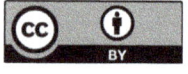

© 2019 by the authors. Licensee MDPI, Basel, Switzerland. This article is an open access article distributed under the terms and conditions of the Creative Commons Attribution (CC BY) license (http://creativecommons.org/licenses/by/4.0/).

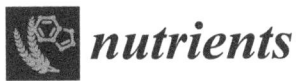

Review

Possible Involvement of Vitamin C in Periodontal Disease-Diabetes Mellitus Association

Maria Bogdan [1,†], Andreea Daniela Meca [1,†], Mihail Virgil Boldeanu [2,*], Dorin Nicolae Gheorghe [3], Adina Turcu-Stiolica [4], Mihaela-Simona Subtirelu [4], Lidia Boldeanu [5], Mihaela Blaj [6,*], Gina Eosefina Botnariu [7], Cristiana Elena Vlad [7], Liliana Georgeta Foia [8] and Petra Surlin [3]

1. Department of Pharmacology, University of Medicine and Pharmacy, 200349 Craiova, Romania; bogdanfmaria81@yahoo.com (M.B.); andreea_mdc@yahoo.com (A.D.M.)
2. Department of Immunology, University of Medicine and Pharmacy, 200349 Craiova, Romania
3. Department of Periodontology, University of Medicine and Pharmacy, 200349 Craiova, Romania; dorinngheorghe@gmail.com (D.N.G.); surlinpetra@gmail.com (P.S.)
4. Department of Pharmacoeconomics, University of Medicine and Pharmacy, 200349 Craiova, Romania; adina.turcu@gmail.com (A.T.-S.); mihaela.subtirelu@yahoo.com (M.-S.S.)
5. Department of Microbiology, University of Medicine and Pharmacy, 200349 Craiova, Romania; barulidia@yahoo.com
6. Department of Surgery, University of Medicine and Pharmacy "Gr. T. Popa", 700115 Iasi, Romania
7. Department of Internal Medicine, University of Medicine and Pharmacy "Gr. T. Popa", 700115 Iasi, Romania; ginabotnariu66@gmail.com (G.E.B.); vladcristiana@gmail.com (C.E.V.)
8. Department of Biochemistry, University of Medicine and Pharmacy "Gr. T. Popa", 700115 Iasi, Romania; lilifoia@yahoo.co.uk
* Correspondence: boldeanumihailvirgil@yahoo.com (M.V.B.); miblaj@yahoo.com (M.B.)
† These authors contributed equally to this work and should be considered first authors

Received: 1 February 2020; Accepted: 17 February 2020; Published: 20 February 2020

Abstract: Ascorbic acid (vitamin C) is an important water-soluble vitamin found in many fruits and vegetables. It has well-documented beneficial effects on the human body and is used as a supplement, alone or in combination with other vitamins and minerals. Over recent years, research has focused on possible new therapeutic actions in chronic conditions including periodontal disease (PD). We conducted a systematic review on clinical trials from four databases (PubMed, Clinical Trials, Cochrane, Web of Science) which measured plasmatic/salivary levels of ascorbic acid in PD–diabetes mellitus (DM) association. Six studies were included in our review, three of them analyzing patients with different grades of PD and DM who received vitamin C as a treatment (500 mg vitamin C/day for 2 months and 450 mg/day for 2 weeks) or as part of their alimentation (guava fruits), in combination with standard therapies and procedures. Decreased levels of vitamin C were observed in PD patients with DM but data about efficacy of vitamin C administration are inconclusive. Given the important bidirectional relationship between PD and DM, there is a strong need for more research to assess the positive effects of ascorbic acid supplementation in individuals suffering from both diseases and also its proper regimen for these patients.

Keywords: vitamin C; ascorbic acid; diabetes mellitus; periodontal disease

1. Introduction

1.1. Diabetes Mellitus, Periodontal Disease and Their Interaction

Diabetes mellitus (DM) is a chronic metabolic disease that alters the physiologic circuit of glucose. If left untreated it can lead to deadly complications such as cardiovascular disease, brain stroke, loss of sight or renal insufficiency. In order to enter a cell and to be used for metabolic purposes, glucose requires the presence of insulin. The pancreas produces insulin, but in some situations, it does not produce enough [1]. This is the cause of type I diabetes, also known as "insulin-dependent DM" because patients need insulin administration during treatment. In other situations, the cells may be resistant and insensitive to insulin action, therefore preventing glucose metabolism. This happens in type II diabetes, which is often associated with obesity. The first stages of type II diabetes treatment include diet control, exercise, and antidiabetic medication but may eventually lead to insulin administration as well. Type II DM is the most common type of adult diabetes, being diagnosed in about 90% of diabetes cases [1].

Periodontal disease (PD) is a chronic inflammatory disorder and a worldwide public health challenge. Since the 1960s scientific evidence has been published regarding an association between DM and periodontitis [2]. It is related to many other chronic diseases, such as cardiovascular disease, inflammatory bowel disease, rheumatoid arthritis, respiratory tract infection and Alzheimer's disease, displaying a particular interest in the relationship between oral and systemic health [3–5]. PD is caused by specific oral microorganisms, such as *Porphyromonas gingivalis*, *Treponema denticola*, *Tannerella forsythia* and *Aggregatibacter actinomycetemcomitans* [6–8], inducing loss of periodontal ligament and alveolar bone, also representing the primary cause of tooth loss [9]. Periodontal impairment is influenced by many risk factors, including alcohol, stress, smoking, heredity, DM and endocrinological changes (pregnancy or menopause); thus, maintaining periodontal health becomes a real challenge [10]. The human oral microbiome is important in the pathogenesis of PD, nutrition being a significant aspect in promoting periodontal homeostasis through antioxidant and immunomodulatory effects on bone metabolism [10–12].

Since 2012, the American Diabetes Association has been including the periodontal examination of diabetic patients in its "Standards of Medical Care for Diabetes". This action has been motivated by the fact that PD was officially recognized as a complication of DM, together with the five other vascular-derived ones (retinopathy, neuropathy, etc.) [13].

Conversely, DM is also credited with an important influence on the pathogenesis process of certain types of PD, as illustrated by the latest classification of periodontal conditions, issued by the European Federation of Periodontology and the American Academy of Periodontology in 2018 [14]. The bidirectional relationship between the two disorders is currently well documented, opening perspectives of common management of diabetic and periodontal patients, in terms of prevention, early diagnosis and integrated treatment protocols [15].

The negative impact that diabetic pathology has on the periodontal status of affected patients has been explained by various mechanisms. From a cellular perspective, it seems that the mobility, activity and efficiency of immune cells, such as polymorphonuclear leukocytes is decreased in a diabetic setting, favoring the aggressive actions of periodontal bacterial pathogens [16,17]. Also, the antibacterial capacity of the saliva and gingival crevicular fluid (GCF) could be downregulated in DM patients, further enhancing the growth of harmful bacteria. In addition to this, periodontal ligament fibroblasts have been shown to decrease chemotaxis when placed in vitro in a hyperglycemic environment [18]. The glucose-rich GCF of DM patients is one such environment, which may explain the difficult periodontal wound healing and the reduced local host response to bacterial attack, all favoring the onset of periodontal inflammation and damage.

Proinflammatory markers, which drive the inflammatory reaction, are secreted by certain immune cells when they are stimulated by bacterial antigens. It has been shown that the immune cells of DM patients over-react to bacterial antigen stimulation, causing an overproduction of proinflammatory markers. Consequently, a more intense inflammatory periodontal reaction is triggered in DM patients, causing the rapid destruction of periodontal tissues [19,20]. The involved proinflammatory markers include major cytokines, such as interleukin 1β (IL-1β), tumor necrosis factor-alpha (TNF-α) and prostaglandin E2 (PGE2), which are all majorly upregulated in DM patients' GCF compared to non-DM patients. When compared, the GCF levels of PGE2 and IL–1β were higher in DM patients' samples than in non-DM ones, in similar settings of PD inflammation and dissolution.

Poorly controlled diabetes is a key factor in the onset of aggressive and destructive forms of PD [21].

Some studies support the direct connection between high PD prevalence and severity in DM patients [22]. This seems to be especially true for type 2 DM patients, who are more prone to difficulty in glycemic control [23]. Poor glycemic control can also impact the outcome of periodontal treatment. Patients with well-controlled glycemia have been shown to reach similar results after nonsurgical periodontal treatment (scaling and root planning) as those of non-DM patients at a four month recall [24]. In contrast, a less favorable response to treatment can be expected from DM patients with uncontrolled glycemia [25]. Periodontal surgery also delivers similar results in terms of periodontal pocket reduction for well-controlled glycemia DM patients compared to non-diabetic ones [26]. Therefore, favorable results can be expected when treating periodontally compromised DM patients with stable glycemia levels.

It was also found that PD patients with undiagnosed DM exhibit significantly increased glycosylated hemoglobin (HbA1C) serum levels compared to periodontally healthy individuals, and PD was positively correlated with serum levels of (HbA1C) before DM onset [27]. If PD acts as an aggravating cofactor for later DM complications, its treatment may be a way to improve the diabetic status and to stabilize glycemic levels, thereby preventing the onset of dangerous complications.

1.2. Oxidative Stress and Reactive Oxygen Species—Background

Oxidative stress is a state of imbalance between oxidants and antioxidants in favor of oxidants, leading to harmful effects [28]. Oxidants, also called reactive oxygen species (ROS), include free radicals such as $O_2 \bullet -$ (superoxide), $ONOO^-$ (peroxynitrite) and $HO \bullet$ (hydroxyl) and nonradicals, such as H_2O_2 (hydrogen peroxide), are products of aerobic cell metabolism by reducing oxygen molecules [29]. There are many sources of ROS, mainly generated by enzymes such as xanthine oxidase, cyclooxygenase, lipooxygenase, myeloperoxidase, cytochrome P450 monooxygenase, uncoupled nitric oxide synthase (NOS), peroxidase and nicotinamide adenine dinucleotide phosphate (NADPH) oxidase. They arise intracellularly, extracellularly, or in specific intracellular compartments [30] and are generated by polymorphonuclear lymphocytes through NADPH oxidase [31].

Oxygen-derived free radicals are oxidative agents produced during events such as mitochondrial respiration and phagocytosis, causing post-translational modifications of proteins, with an impact on cell signaling, gene expression and other physiological processes [32]. Low concentrations of ROS enhance antioxidant response by activating a nuclear factor erythroid 2-related factor 2, promoting cell survival [33]. ROS-induced impairment of glycocalyx, cell membranes and junctions contribute to increased permeability and leukocyte and thrombocyte adhesion, with subsequent local activation of inflammation and coagulation, leading to loss of endothelial vasodilation potential and attenuation of vasoconstrictor response [34].

There is also a documented link between oxidative stress, DM and PD, with the oxidative-stress-mediated changes in the inflammatory pathways being possible mechanisms in affecting periodontal tissues [35] (Figure 1). DM and PD involve significant impairment of immune system regulation, while hyperglycemia contributes to advanced glycation end products (AGE) formation and extended levels of proinflammatory cytokines IL-1β, interleukin 6 (IL-6) and TNF-α [36] (Figure 1).

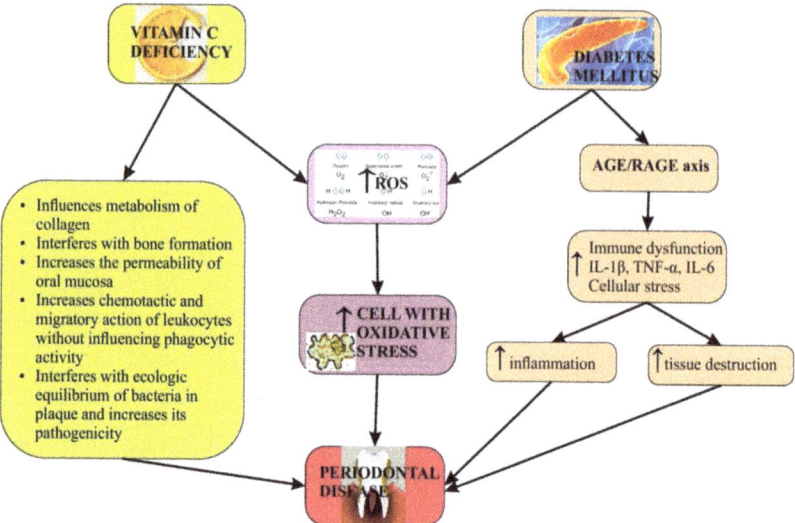

Figure 1. The interrelation between vitamin C, diabetes mellitus (DM) and periodontal disease (PD).

1.3. Vitamin C, DM, and PD

In the 1920s, the forthcoming Nobel laureate Albert Szent-Györgyi from Szeged University, Hungary, identified vitamin C and its role in preventing and treating scurvy [37]. Ascorbic acid (vitamin C) is an essential water-soluble vitamin that cannot be synthesized by the human organism [38,39]. It demands a regular and appropriate intake from natural sources, like citrus fruits, mango, strawberries, kiwi, papaya, green leafy vegetables, tomatoes and broccoli [37], to hamper hypovitaminosis C that is relatively common in Western populations [38,39].

Synthetic vitamin C derived from chemicals is similar to that contained in fruits and vegetables [40]. The main route of administration for ascorbic acid is oral ingestion from food or supplements. Healthy individuals generally need 0.1–0.2 g daily doses. Intravenous administration is used in critically ill patients requiring high doses (1–4 g/day) of this nutrient [41,42]. It is quickly eliminated by the kidneys with a half-life of approximately two hours [41,43].

L-ascorbate, the reduced form of vitamin C, is a physiological antioxidant [44]. Antioxidants are molecules that can donate a hydrogen atom or an electron to a radical, ceasing chain reactions [45] such as metal chelation and protecting cells from radiation damage and the formation of nonradical and nonreactive end products of antioxidant enzymes [28].

Vitamin C improves immune function and facilitates iron absorption, reduction of folic acid derivatives and synthesis of collagen, cortisol, catecholamines and carnitine [46]. Vitamin C also improves the synthesis of prostaglandins PGE1 and PGI2 and nitric oxide (eNO); it has a cytoprotection role, antimutagenic activity, vasodilatory action and inhibitory effect on platelet aggregation, being useful in type 2 DM and high blood pressure [47].

Ascorbic acid deficiency has been associated with stroke, DM, cancer, cardiovascular disease, infectious diseases and sepsis [41].

In type 2 DM the plasma levels of IL-6 and TNF-α are elevated, lipid peroxides are increased and unsaturated fatty acids, especially arachidonic acid (AA) and lipoxin A4 (LXA4), are reduced [48]. Besides, the usefulness of vitamin C in the management of type 2 DM is confirmed by a study conducted by Mason et al. [49] which recorded that oral vitamin C (1000 mg daily) reduced hyperglycemia. This action arose after a decrease of plasma isoprostane-F2 in these subjects and indicated that the beneficial action of vitamin C was not only due to its antioxidant property but also to its ability to improve PGE1, PGI2, LXA4 and eNO [49].

Oxidative stress plays an important role in the development of vascular complications in type 2 DM, and the increase of ROS level is due to decreased production of some enzymatic/nonenzymatic antioxidants, i.e., catalase, superoxide dismutase (SOD) and glutathione peroxidase (GSH-Px), leading to the development of diabetic complications [50]. Free radical formation in type 2 DM is accomplished by nonenzymatic proteins glycation, oxidation of glucose, increased lipid peroxidation, inducing enzyme damage and increased insulin resistance [51]. Insulin signaling is modulated by ROS/RNS (reactive nitrogen species) in two ways: first, in response to insulin, ROS/RNS exerts a physiological function; second, the ROS and RNS pathway negatively regulates insulin signaling, contributing to development of insulin resistance, which is a risk factor for type 2 DM [52].

Oxidative stress and ROS induce complications of DM including coronary heart disease, neuropathy, nephropathy, retinopathy and stroke [50]. Hyperglycemia plays a role in the generation of oxidative stress leading to vascular endothelial dysfunction of patients with DM and, together with dyslipidemia, develops macroangiopathies, which cause oxidative stress leading to atherosclerosis [50]. Vitamin C acts as an antioxidant by detoxification of ROS, hence being an important biomarker of oxidative stress, but, depending on the situation, it might promote toxicity via pro-oxidant formation [51].

Vitamin C plays a key role in maintaining the integrity of the connective tissues, thus of the periodontium. It is a powerful antioxidant, particularly at the intracellular level, being an enzymatic cofactor in metabolic reactions (hydroxylation of proline and lysine needed to stabilize collagen structures during its synthesis) [10].

Regarding the interplay between vitamin C and PD, the results of observational studies are contradictory, depending on the parameter evaluated, with several studies reporting no association between vitamin C and PD [10]. However, Nishida et al. [53] in their study with 12,419 participants identified a dose-dependent relationship between the vitamin C intake and the number of people with PD. Contrary to these results, a relation between vitamin C deficiency and PD was not recorded by other researches [54,55].

Vitamin C intake is necessary to avoid periodontal issues, but when a pathological condition has been established, a supplement with vitamin C is not sufficient to cure periodontal pathology [10]. Also, the effect of vitamin C combined with chlorhexidine can prevent and slow down the PD progression [56].

Monea et al. [57], in a case-control study (which included 10 patients with type 2 DM and 8 healthy adults), observed significantly increased malondialdehyde (MDA) levels in periodontal tissues, suggesting increased lipid peroxidation and decreased glutathione tissue levels (GSH), resulting a change of the local defense mechanism. Thus, histological aspects in the periodontal tissues of diabetic subjects confirm the involvement of oxidative stress [57].

In a study with murine models with diabetes, Li et al. [58] found that simultaneous periodontitis and DM synergistically aggravated both local and systemic oxidative lesions, being correlated with more severe periodontal destruction in diabetic periodontitis.

In a study with 10,930 patients, Lee et al. [59] found that in patients with DM between the ages of 30 and 49, there was a significant link between vitamin C intake and periodontitis. In the stratified analysis, the aforementioned association was highlighted among patients with type 2 DM. When there was inadequate vitamin C intake, diabetic subjects were more sensitive to oxidative stress, developing PD. These results pointed out the crucial role of vitamin C in promoting periodontal health among adults [59].

In a prospective cohort study that included 579 men, Dietrich et al. [60] observed that participants with periodontitis had a lower intake of vitamin C, increased risk of DM, higher levels of bleeding, bacterial plaque, loss of attachment and fewer teeth.

Considering the positive association between PD and ischemic heart disease, serum and salivary levels of vitamin C were analyzed in patients suffering from both conditions and were found to be lower compared to PD patients and healthy individuals [61].

The present study aims to systematically review the available clinical data about the plasmatic and salivary levels of ascorbic acid in patients affected by PD and DM and about possible beneficial effects of ascorbic acid supplementation in PD–DM association.

2. Methods

The protocol of the review was developed following the Preferred Reporting Items for Systematic Reviews and Meta-Analyses (PRISMA) statement guidelines [62] and was designed to gather the results of clinical trials in patients with different grades of PD and DM whose plasma levels of vitamin C were determined.

2.1. Study Selection Criteria

The population of interest for this review included patients with a current diagnosis of both chronic PD and DM (type 1 or type 2). All the studies which met the following inclusion criteria were included in this systematic review: (1) written in English; (2) published before 8 September 2019; (3) investigating association between vitamin C, PD and DM; (4) clinical trials conducted on adults; and (5) using quantitative methods of data collection. The design of the targeted studies, which were of interest, depended on the dosage and frequency of administration of ascorbic acid, both as therapeutic administration and as part of the patients' usual alimentation. Other types of studies, such as cohort, randomized and cross-sectional surveys were also included. Studies that included only plasmatic or salivary measurements of vitamin C were also of interest and included. Articles' exclusion criteria were: (1) written in a language other than English; (2) reviews and animal studies; (3) abstract only or no abstract; (4) not mentioning whether the patients had DM or not; or (5) not measuring ascorbic acid plasma/salivary levels.

2.2. Literature Search

The electronic literature search was conducted by two independent authors (M.B. and A.D.M.) within the following databases: PubMed, Clinical Trials, Cochrane and Web of Science.

The inclusion criteria were defined according to the PICO model: population (P = "human adults"), intervention or exposure (I = "impact of vitamin C on patients with PD and DM"), comparison (C = "dosage and frequency of dosage for vitamin C, received as treatment or as part of alimentation; different concentrations of plasmatic vitamin C"), and outcome (O = "measurement of periodontal status using specific disease parameters"). The following PICO question was used: "Is vitamin C associated with an improvement of periodontal status in patients with DM?"

Four types of searches in each database were performed with the exact term combination: type 1—"vitamin C AND periodontal disease AND diabetes mellitus" OR type 2—"ascorbic acid AND periodontal disease AND diabetes mellitus" OR type 3—"vitamin C AND periodontitis AND diabetes mellitus" OR type 4—"ascorbic acid AND periodontitis AND diabetes mellitus".

2.3. Selection of Studies

Both authors assessed the eligibility of all the studies and screened them, eliminating duplicates and removing all the studies that did not respect the selection criteria after assessing the content from titles and abstracts. The reviewers shared their independently obtained data and resolved decided any disagreements by general approval. The final titles were included for further data extraction and analysis.

2.4. Data Extraction and Analysis

The two authors independently extracted data from the final articles into an Excel template developed by the research team. The included elements were publication year, study type design, the country where the study was run, participants' characteristics (number, age and gender), periodontal status and type of measurement, type of intervention, along with diabetes status and type of measurement. The experimental design of the final list of studies was reported to cover the duration of the study, the administration (dosage and frequency) of vitamin C, the measurement of vitamin C and their main results.

3. Results

The literature search resulted in 71 articles across the four databases (PubMed, Clinical Trials, Cochrane, Web of Science), of which 33 were reviewed after duplicates (n = 38) were removed (Figure 2). After screening with inclusion/exclusion criteria, six papers remained for the systematic analysis. Detailed summaries of final studies are included in Tables 1 and 2.

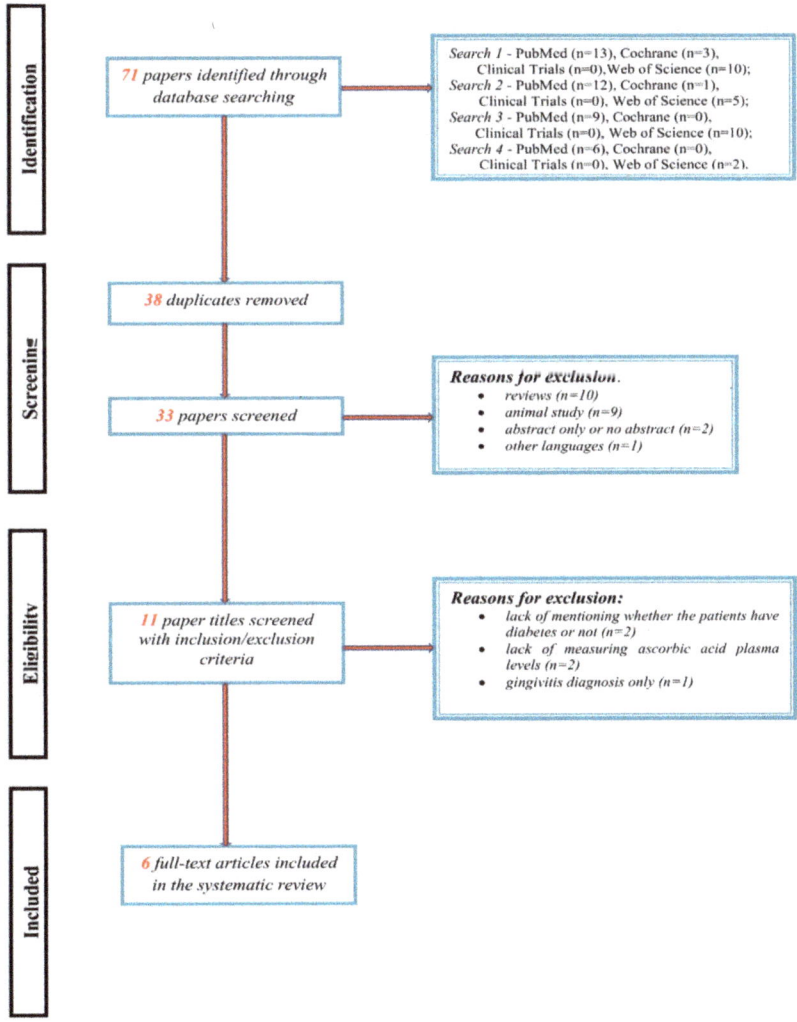

Figure 2. Flowchart of the systematic search based on PRISMA guidelines.

Table 1. General data of the eligible studies.

Reference	Study Type	Country	Participant Characteristics (Study Sample)			Periodontal Status	Measurement of Periodontal Status	Intervention	Diabetes Status	Measurement of Diabetes
			No.	Age	Gender					
Gumus, 2009 [66]	CC	Turkey	65	17–73 years old	M and F	16 patients with type 1 DM (5 M, 11F, age: 17–73), 25 patients with type 2 (11 M, 14F, age: 42–69) and 24 systematically healthy (control group, 10 M, 14 F, age: 22–60), all with PD	plaque-induced inflammatory PD, non-aggressive. PII, PB, gingival recession, CAL, BOP, recorded for 6 sites per tooth.	full-mouth periodontal clinical measurements	type 1 or type 2	FBS, HbA1C, and diabetes complications
Thomas, 2010 [65]	CC	India	60	adults	M and F	3 groups: group 1—20 patients with type 2 DM and PD, group 2—20 healthy patients with PD and group 3—20 healthy patients without PD	CAL measured with a Williams periodontal probe and BOP	examinations	type 2	RBS, FBS
Gokhale, 2013 [63]	RS	India	120	30–60 years old	M and F	4 groups of 30 patients each group 1: no PD, group 2: chronic gingivitis, group 3: chronic periodontitis, group 4: chronic periodontitis and recently diagnosed type 2 diabetes; randomized subjects of groups 2–4, were grouped to receive SRP with dietary supplementation of ascorbic acid for 2 weeks or only SRP; chronic periodontitis—PPD and assessment of gingival bleeding	PII, SBI for gingivitis, PPDs for chronic periodontitis, gingival bleeding	randomized subjects within groups 2–4, divided to receive either SRP or not	type 2	CPC, FBS, PPG
Amaliya, 2015 [68]	CH	Indonesia	98	39–50 years old	45 M and 53 F	remote populations deprived of oral health care—natural development of periodontitis; subjects of this population showed a mean of 30% ABL in their dentition, ranging from 19% to 54%	dental radiographs, ABL, periapical radiologic transparency	examinations	a small number of subjects (70% in prediabetic state and 6% having undiagnosed diabetes) with HbA1c values ≥6.5%	HbA1C
Patil, 2016 [67]	CS	India	100	adults	M and F	4 groups: 25 normal healthy controls, 25 gingivitis patients, 25 chronic periodontitis patients, 25 chronic periodontitis and type 2 diabetes	BOP, SBI, PPD	examinations	type 2	FBS, PPG
Kunsongkeit, 2019 [64]	Double-blind, placebo-controlled, clinical trial	Thailand	31	43–72 years old	9 M and 22 F	moderate chronic periodontitis, 2 groups: n = 15 who received periodontal therapy and vitamin C for 2 months and n = 16 who received periodontal therapy and placebo	PII, SBI, gingival index, PPD	full SRP and examinations	type 2 uncontrolled (FBS > 150 mg/dL, HbA1c > 7%)	FBS, HbA1C

Abbreviations (in alphabetical order): ABL—alveolar bone loss, BOP—bleeding on probing, CAL—clinical attachment level, CC—case-control study, CH—cohort study, CPC—casual plasma glucose, CS—cross-sectional survey, DM—diabetes mellitus, FBS—fasting blood sugar, LS—longitudinal study, PB—probing depth, PII—plaque index, PD—periodontal disease, PPDs—probing pocket depths, PPG—two-hour postprandial glucose, RBS—random blood sugar, ROS—reactive species of oxygen, RS—randomized study, SBI—sulcus bleeding index, SRP—scaling and root planning.

Table 2. Experimental design.

Reference	Duration	Dosage	Administration	Frequency	Measurement of Vitamin C	Main Results
Gumus, 2009 [66]	2 and 1/2 years	none	none	none	measurement of antioxidants' salivary concentrations in whole saliva samples	Subjects with type 2 DM had fewer teeth and more sites with probing depths (>4 mm) than patients with type 1 DM. Despite this, total antioxidant capacity and vitamin C concentrations did not seem to play a major role in the pathogenesis of periodontitis correlated with DM.
Thomas, 2010 [65]	Not mentioned	none	none	none	venous blood samples collected	Diabetic patients with periodontitis revealed a significant decrease in vitamin C levels.
Gokhale, 2013 [63]	4 months	450 mg	subgroups randomly divided using a coin-toss method: subgroup A (15) 450 mg chewable tablet and subgroup B (15) placebo chewable tablet	daily intake for 2 weeks or only SRP	plasma measurement	Plasma measured AAL were below the normal range in systemically healthy subjects with gingivitis and diabetics with periodontitis. Dietary AA supplementation associated with SRP improved the SBI in patients with gingivitis and PD-DM.
Amaliya, 2015 [68]	1 year	food products categorized as high (>60 mg), fair (31–60 mg), low (2–30 mg) or no vitamin C (<2 mg vitamin C/100 g)	Number of guava fruit servings	food frequency taken in the last month	plasma measurement, based on the values provided by the National Nutrient Database for standard reference	45% of the participants showed vitamin C depletion/deficiency, 70% were in a prediabetic state, 6% had untreated diabetes. Still, it has been shown that guava fruit consumption might have played a protective role against periodontitis in a malnourished population, regarding the extent and severity of ABL (at least 10% of the participants had a low BMI and were considered as malnourished).
Patil, 2016 [67]	1 year	none	none	none	plasma measurement	A significant decrease in vitamin C was observed in the diabetic periodontitis group as compared with healthy control groups. Type 2 diabetic subjects revealed excessive ROS concentration, therefore more periodontal tissue destruction.
Kunsongkeit, 2019 [64]	2 months	500 mg	tablets	daily for 2 months	plasma measurement	Periodontitis patients with uncontrolled type 2 DM did not have evident benefits by supplementation of 500 mg/day vitamin C.

Abbreviations (in alphabetical order): ABL—alveolar bone loss, AA—ascorbic acid, AAL—ascorbic acid levels, BMI—body mass index, DM—diabetes mellitus, PB—probing depth, PPDs—probing pocket depths, ROS—reactive species of oxygen, SBI—sulcus bleeding index, SRP—scaling and root planning.

Two of the remaining six studies aimed to evaluate the relationship between plasma ascorbic acid levels and PD in systemically healthy and type 2 DM subjects, following the administration of vitamin C in similar 450–500 mg daily doses. Gokhale et al. [63] randomly divided participants into subgroups, using a coin-toss method: subgroup A (15 adults) receiving 450 mg chewable tablet associated with daily scaling and root planning and subgroup B (15 adults) receiving placebo as lemon-flavored sugar-free candy chewable tablets with scaling and root planning spaced over two appointments. It revealed that dietary ascorbic acid supplementation associated with scaling and root planning improved the sulcus bleeding index in subjects with gingivitis and diabetics with periodontitis. They also obtained additional results, by using Tukey's multiple post-hoc procedures, regarding the plasma ascorbic acid levels in subgroup A, which supported their conclusion [63]. Similarly, Kunsongkeit et al. [64] assessed the administration of daily 500 mg vitamin C tablets, for 2 months in 15 adults or placebo tablets in 16 adults, both groups receiving full scaling and root planning from baseline to the last administered tablet, comparing the results within groups using Bonferroni post-hoc test. Periodontitis patients with uncontrolled type 2 DM did not exhibit evident benefits by supplementation of 500 mg/day vitamin C [64], but the differences between their results may have been generated by the recently diagnosed type 2 DM patients included in the Gokhale et al. study and uncontrolled type 2 DM patients included in the Kunsongkeit el al. study. Therefore, the progression and severity of periodontitis were greater in patients with uncontrolled diabetes and perhaps the dosage of vitamin C should have been larger to sustain the conclusions revealed in the Gokhale et al. study. Even so, both studies assumed the bidirectional relationship between periodontitis and DM, which means further assessments should be aimed by other medical specialists.

Three studies from the ones selected [65–67] evaluated the effect of dietary intake of vitamin C, as an antioxidant and immunomodulatory agent, and the evolution of PD in patients with DM, without specifying certain consumed fruits or vegetables or dosage, but measuring plasmatic [65,67] or salivary concentration of ascorbic acid [66]. Thomas et al. [65] measured plasmatic ascorbic acid levels in their case-control study by using spectrophotometric quantitation on all three groups: 20 patients with type 2 DM and PD, 20 healthy patients with PD and 20 healthy patients without PD. This method was useful for comparing the micronutrient levels not only of vitamin C but also of zinc and copper in diabetic patients and healthy individuals with periodontitis, finally showing that diet plays a modifying role in the progression of periodontal disease. The idea was sustained by a statistically significant decrease in vitamin C levels in diabetic patients with periodontitis when compared to healthy individuals with periodontitis [65]. The same conclusion appeared in a cross-sectional survey, also held in India, by Patil et al. [67], even though vitamin C was measured by a different chemical method (dinitro phenyl hydrazine method). They included an additional group consisting of patients who suffered from gingivitis, an incipient form of PD, and a group of recently diagnosed patients who suffered from periodontitis and diabetes, who had not received any antidiabetic medication, before the study onset [67]. Gumus et al. [66] conducted a case-control study in Turkey by measuring the total antioxidant capacity in patients with PD, divided into three groups: 16 patients with type 1 DM, 25 patients with type 2 DM and 24 patients with no associated disease. They used the Kruskal–Wallis test, followed by the Mann–Whitney U test for the group comparisons of the salivary antioxidant levels, as well as the clinical periodontal measurements; however, their conclusion was different from the Indian studies, because vitamin C did not seem to play a major role in the pathogenesis of periodontal manifestations in diabetes. They mentioned the absence of a group with diabetes with a clinically healthy periodontium which would have enabled them to conclude whether the levels of salivary antioxidants are related to the diabetic status independently of the clinical periodontal situation [66]. This limitation of the Turkish study might have led to a different conclusion regarding the ascorbic acid levels in patients with both diabetes and periodontitis than the one commonly presented in Indian studies.

Amaliya et al. [68] organized a cohort study in Indonesia analyzing the intake of vitamin C from the dietary origin while monitoring all 98 patients using a full set of dental radiographs with long cone paralleling technique. Their results depended on the consumption of guava fruit over one month in all 53 women and 45 men, with an age range from 39 to 50 years, who were included in the study. Amaliya et al. stated that guava fruit contains 228 mg vitamin C per 100 g (USDA 2010), which implied that the consumption of one guava (without skin and kernel) results in an intake of about 400 mg vitamin C. Since the guava consumption varied between 0 and 30 guavas in the month preceding plasmatic ascorbic acid measurements, a great variation in the amount of vitamin C intake existed in their included population, possibly contributing to the significant association with alveolar bone loss. In their study, 45% of the population showed vitamin C depletion/deficiency, 70% were in a prediabetic state and 6% had untreated diabetes. Their new finding was that guava fruit consumption may play a protective role against periodontitis in the 10% malnourished population, which showed a relatively low body mass index. These conditions may have contributed to the extent and severity of alveolar bone loss in the population. It is important to mention that Amaliya et al. had a limitation because 70% of their population were in a prediabetic state and 6% had undiagnosed diabetes, which is why no relation could be assessed between HbA1c plasma levels and alveolar bone loss, probably due to the small number of subjects with HbA1c values ≥6.5% and insufficient conclusive data of the study [68].

All studies included in our systematic review had in common the assessment indication for PD, which included certain parameters: alveolar bone loss, bleeding on probing, clinical attachment level (CAL > 3 mm), the community periodontal index, pocket depth or probing pocket depths (PPDs of ≥5 mm, along with the presence of attachment loss of ≥2 mm within at least three teeth (assessed at four sites per tooth)), plaque index and the sulcus bleeding index (SBI score of ≥2).

The plaque index had the following scoring criteria: score 0—no plaque, score 1—a film of plaque adhering to the free gingival margin and the adjacent area of the tooth, seen in situ only after the application of disclosure solution or by using the probe on the tooth surface, score 2—moderate accumulation of soft deposits within the gingival pocket, or the tooth and gingival margin, which can be seen with the naked eye, score 3—abundance of soft matter within the gingival pocket and/or on the tooth and gingival margin [63]. The assessment of gingival bleeding is done on a scale of 0–5 according to the following criteria: score 0—healthy appearance of the gingiva and no bleeding upon sulcus probing, score 1—apparently healthy gingiva showing no color or contour changes and no swelling, but sulcus bleeding on probing, score 2—bleeding on probing and color change caused by inflammation, but absent swelling, score 3—bleeding on probing, change in color and slight edematous swelling, score 4—bleeding on probing, obvious color change and swelling, and score 5—spontaneous bleeding on probing, color change, marked swelling with or without ulceration [63].

The parameters used to sustain the diagnosis of DM included body mass index (BMI), glycosylated hemoglobin (HbA1C > 7%), fasting blood sugar (FBS ≥ 126 mg/dL), two-hour postprandial glucose (PPG ≥ 200 mg/dL) and random blood sugar (RBS ≥ 200 mg/dL with symptoms such as polyuria, polydipsia and polyphagia).

4. Discussions

Three of our selected studies [63,65,67] were held in India, with a similar number of participants (60–120) and similarly composed groups of study, classified by periodontal status, but with the first two not mentioning their age. All the Indian studies used plasmatic measurement of vitamin C and they also had in common a finding regarding the lower plasmatic levels of ascorbic acid in periodontitis and diabetic patients than periodontitis nondiabetic patients. Four of our six eligible studies [63–65,67] excluded patients with any systemic disorder (other than the groups with type 1 or type 2 DM), those with presence of any disease that may alter the immune system (bacterial or viral infections, hypercholesterolemia, cardiovascular events), those who had been treated with any dietary supplements, antibiotics, and anti-inflammatory drugs in the previous 6 months, those with history of smoking or tobacco consumption, those with history of using any mechanical or chemical aids for plaque control (mouthwashes) and pregnant subjects. On the other hand, two studies included smokers (for example, Gumus et al. [66] recorded patients' smoking history), one of them targeting the smoking population to shape a conclusion (Amaliya et al. [68] included 26 heavy smokers of which the number of cigarettes per day ranged from 15 to 24 and 19 light smokers who smoked on average 8 cigarettes per day), but fulfilled the other exclusion criteria present in all the mentioned studies.

An interesting conclusion was presented in Amaliya et al.'s [68] study, referring to vitamin C as an important prophylactic and protective measure, especially in malnourished people with both DM and PD, even though they included heavy smokers with high exposure to ROS. Their results were based on the intake of about 400 mg vitamin C daily, for at least one month, by consuming approximately 30 guava fruits, a specific diet for people living in Purbasari Tea Estate in West Java, Indonesia [68]. On the contrary, Gumus et al. only supported a difference between diabetic patients regarding the evolution of PD by mentioning that subjects with type 2 DM had fewer teeth and more sites with probing depths >4 mm than patients with type 1 DM. In this study, vitamin C and the total antioxidant capacity did not appear to play a significant role in the pathogenesis of PD–DM [66].

Individuals afflicted with DM and PD may also exhibit a decrease in vitamin C concentration through a confounding factor, depression. Depression often complicates the management of other conditions (cancer, diabetes, myocardial infarction, severe trauma) or can occur secondary to other diseases such as inflammatory conditions, Parkinson's disease and hypothyroidism [69].

Some articles demonstrated the association between poor vitamin C and increased depression symptoms [70,71], between DM and depression [72] and between severe PD [73] and depression. Studies have shown that depression is a consequence of inadequate levels of ascorbic acid [74]. More, vitamin C can reduce the problems associated with depression [75]. Depression prevalence is two to three times higher in patients with DM, with some cases remaining underdiagnosed [76]. Depression is also a risk factor for PD [77–79]. This is the reason some future research must be done to minimize the influence of this confounding factor and evaluate its strength using different questionnaires [80,81].

Several recent reviews analyzed the role of vitamin C in the pathophysiology of periodontal tissue damage [10,54,82,83].

Kaur et al. and Muniz et al. pointed out the beneficial effects of ascorbic acid as a dietary antioxidant on PD management in the context of the established link between PD and oxidative stress. They implied that, as a complementary treatment for PD, the use of an antioxidant has the potential to improve periodontal clinical parameters [82,83].

In 2018, Varela-Lopez et al. [10] performed a systematic review of human and animal studies, and they concluded that vitamin C may be useful for prevention or improvement of PD. They also emphasized the need for more research to clarify dosages and taking frequency of ascorbic acid supplementation.

In a systematic review from 2019, Tada and Miura [54] highlighted the effects of vitamin C on the prevention of incidence and the development of PD. The authors observed proof of the association between vitamin C, PD and DM which suggests a complex mechanism of action between ascorbic acid and the two disorders that requires further study.

In our analysis, decreased levels of vitamin C were observed in PD patients with DM but data about efficacy of vitamin C administration are few and inconclusive. Perhaps larger doses administered over a longer period of time are needed, especially for periodontitis patients with uncontrolled type 2 DM.

To our knowledge, this is the first systematic review to assess and summarize the current outcomes on the correlation between ascorbic acid levels and PD–DM interaction. There are limitations to the present study because of the heterogeneity of the included studies' methodology. The findings of our review reflect different outcomes because of the different experimental designs.

5. Conclusions

Considering the complex and strong relation between DM and PD and the paucity of available clinical evidence for the effects of ascorbic acid in individuals affected by both conditions, further detailed studies should be performed to establish the efficacy of vitamin C for these patients. Besides the issue of the required doses, the frequency and duration of administration for ascorbic acid supplements need to be clarified.

Author Contributions: Conceptualization: M.B. (Maria Bogdan), P.S.; literature research: M.B. (Maria Bogdan), A.D.M.; methodology: A.T.-S., M.-S.S.; writing—original draft: M.B. (Maria Bogdan), A.D.M., C.E.V., D.N.G., L.B.; writing—review and editing: M.V.B., M.B. (Mihaela Blaj), P.S.; supervision: L.G.F., G.E.B. All authors have read and agreed to the published version of the manuscript.

Funding: This research received no external funding.

Conflicts of Interest: The authors declare no conflict of interest.

References

1. American Diabetes Association. Diagnosis and classification of diabetes mellitus. *Diabetes Care* **2013**, *36* (Suppl. S1), S67–S74.
2. Liccardo, D.; Cannavo, A.; Spagnuolo, G.; Ferrara, N.; Cittadini, A.; Rengo, C.; Rengo, G. Periodontal Disease: A Risk Factor for Diabetes and Cardiovascular Disease. *Int. J. Mol. Sci.* **2019**, *20*, 1414. [CrossRef]
3. Van der Velden, U.; Kuzmanova, D.; Chapple, I.L. Micronutritional approaches to periodontal therapy. *J. Clin. Periodontol.* **2011**, *38* (Suppl. S11), 142–158. [CrossRef]
4. Bui, F.Q.; Almeida-da-Silva, C.L.C.; Huynh, B.; Trinh, A.; Liu, J.; Woodward, J.; Asadi, H.; Ojcius, D.M. Association between periodontal pathogens and systemic disease. *Biomed. J.* **2019**, *42*, 27–35. [CrossRef] [PubMed]
5. Martu, M.A.; Solomon, S.M.; Toma, V.; Maftei, G.A.; Iovan, A.; Gamen, A.; Hurjui, L.; Rezus, E.; Foia, L.; Forna, N.C. The importance of cytokines in periodontal disease and rheumatoid arthritis. Review. *Rom. J. Oral Rehabil.* **2019**, *11*, 230–240.
6. How, K.Y.; Song, K.P.; Chan, K.G. Porphyromonasgingivalis: An Overview of Periodontopathic Pathogen below the Gum Line. *Front. Microbiol.* **2016**, *7*, 53. [CrossRef]
7. Mysak, J.; Podzimek, S.; Sommerova, P.; Lyuya-Mi, Y.; Bartova, J.; Janatova, T.; Prochazkova, J.M.; Duskova, J. Porphyromonas gingivalis: major periodontopathic pathogen overview. *J. Immunol. Res.* **2014**, *2014*, 476068. [CrossRef] [PubMed]
8. Belibasakis, G.N.; Maula, T.; Bao, K.; Lindholm, M.; Bostanci, N.; Oscarsson, J.; Ihalin, R.; Johansson, A. Virulence and Pathogenicity Properties of *Aggregatibacteractino mycetemcomitans*. *Pathogens* **2019**, *8*, 222. [CrossRef] [PubMed]
9. Zong, G.; Scott, A.E.; Griffiths, H.R.; Zockm, P.L.; Dietrich, T.; Newson, R.S. Serum alpha-Tocopherol Has a Nonlinear Inverse Association with Periodontitis among US Adults. *J. Nutr.* **2015**, *145*, 893–899. [CrossRef]
10. Varela-Lopez, A.; Navarro-Hortal, M.D.; Giampieri, F.; Bullon, P.; Battino, M.; Quiles, J.L. Nutraceuticals in Periodontal Health: A Systematic Review on the Role of Vitamins in Periodontal Health Maintenance. *Molecules* **2018**, *23*, 1226. [CrossRef]
11. Alagl, A.S.; Bhat, S.G. Ascorbic acid: New role of an age-old micronutrient in the management of periodontal disease in older adults. *Geriatr. Gerontol. Int.* **2015**, *15*, 241–254. [CrossRef] [PubMed]
12. Nasri, H.; Baradaran, A.; Shirzad, H.; Rafieian-Kopaei, M. New concepts in nutraceuticals as alternative for pharmaceuticals. *Int. J. Prev. Med.* **2014**, *5*, 1487–1499. [PubMed]
13. American Diabetes Association. Standards of Medical Care in Diabetes. *Diabetes Care* **2012**, *35*, S11. [CrossRef] [PubMed]
14. Caton, J.; Armitage, G.; Berglundh, T.; Berglundh, T.; Chapple, I.L.C.; Jepsen, S.; Kornman, K.S.; Mealey, B.L.; Papapanou, P.N.; Sanz, M.; et al. A new classification scheme for periodontal and peri-implant diseases and conditions – Introduction and keychanges from the 1999 classification. *J. Clin. Periodontol.* **2018**, *45* (Suppl. S20), S1–S8.
15. Sanz, M.; Ceriello, A.; Buysschaert, M.; Chapple, I.; Demmer, R.T.; Graziani, F.; Herrera, D.; Jepsen, S.; Lione, L.; Madianos, P.; et al. Scientific evidence on the links between periodontal diseases and diabetes: Consensus report and guidelines of the joint workshop on periodontal diseases and diabetes by the International Diabetes Federation and the EuropeanFederation of Periodontology. *J. Clin. Periodontol.* **2018**, *45*, 138–149. [CrossRef]
16. Gurav, A.; Jadhav, V. Periodontitis and risk of diabetes mellitus. *J. Diabetes* **2011**, *3*, 21–28. [CrossRef]

17. Demmer, R.T.; Jacobs, D.R., Jr.; Desvarieux, M. Periodontal disease and incident type 2 diabetes: Results from the First National Health and Nutrition Examination Survey and its epidemiologic follow-up study. *Diabetes Care* **2008**, *31*, 1373–1379. [CrossRef]
18. Huang, J.; Xiao, Y.; Xu, A.; Zhou, Z. Neutrophils in type 1 diabetes. *J. Diabetes Investig.* **2016**, *7*, 652–663. [CrossRef]
19. Olteanu, M.; Surlin, P.; Oprea, B.; Rauten, A.M.; Popescu, R.M.; Nițu, M.; Camen, G.C.; Caraivan, O. Gingival inflammatory infiltrate analysis in patients with chronic periodontitis and diabetes mellitus. *Rom. J. Morphol. Embryol.* **2011**, *52*, 1311–1317.
20. Șurlin, P.; Camen, A.; Stratul, S.I.; Roman, A.; Gheorghe, D.N.; Herăscu, E.; Osiac, E.; Rogoveanu, I. Optical coherence tomography assessment of gingival epithelium inflammatory status in periodontal—Systemic affected patients. *Ann. Anat.* **2018**, *219*, 51–56. [CrossRef]
21. Wendt, T.; Tanji, N.; Guo, J.; Hudson, B.I.; Bierhaus, A.; Ramasamy, R.; Arnold, B.; Nawroth, P.P.; Yan, S.F.; D'Agati, V.; et al. Glucose, glycation, and RAGE: Implications for amplification of cellular dysfunction in diabetic nephropathy. *J. Am. Soc. Nephrol.* **2003**, *14*, 1383–1395. [CrossRef] [PubMed]
22. Rafatjou, R.; Razavi, Z.; Tayebi, S.; Khalili, M.; Farhadian, M. Dental Health Status and Hygiene in Children and Adolescents with Type 1 Diabetes Mellitus. *J. Res. Health Sci.* **2016**, *16*, 122–126. [PubMed]
23. Mirza, B.A.; Syed, A.; Izhar, F.; Ali Khan, A. Bidirectional relationship between diabetes and periodontal disease: Review of evidence. *J. Pak. Med. Assoc.* **2010**, *60*, 766–768. [PubMed]
24. Mizuno, H.; Ekuni, D.; Maruyama, T.; Kataoka, K.; Yoneda, T.; Fukuhara, D.; Sugiura, Y.; Tomofuji, T.; Wada, J.; Morita, M. The effects of non-surgical periodontal treatment on glycemic control, oxidative stress balance and quality of life in patients with type 2 diabetes: A randomized clinical trial. *PLoS ONE* **2017**, *12*, e0188171. [CrossRef] [PubMed]
25. Dağ, A.; Firat, E.T.; Arikan, S.; Kadiroğlu, A.K.; Kaplan, A. The effect of periodontal therapy on serum TNF-alpha and HbA1c levels in type 2 diabetic patients. *Aust. Dent. J.* **2009**, *54*, 17–22. [CrossRef]
26. Li, Q.; Hao, S.; Fang, J.; Xie, J.; Kong, X.H.; Yang, J.X. Effect of non-surgical periodontal treatment on glycemic control of patients with diabetes: A meta-analysis of randomized controlled trials. *Trials* **2015**, *16*, 291. [CrossRef]
27. Isola, G.; Matarese, G.; Ramaglia, L.; Pedullà, E.; Rapisarda, E.; Iorio-Siciliano, V. Association between periodontitis and glycosylated haemoglobin before diabetes onset: A cross-sectional study. *Clin. Oral Investig.* **2019**. [CrossRef]
28. Sies, H. Oxidative stress: Oxidants and antioxidants. *Exp. Physiol.* **1997**, *82*, 291–295. [CrossRef]
29. Ray, R.; Shah, A.M. NADPH oxidase and endothelial cell function. *Clin. Sci.* **2005**, *109*, 217–226. [CrossRef]
30. Griendling, K.K.; FitzGerald, G.A. Oxidative stress and cardiovascular injury: Part I: Basic mechanisms and in vivo monitoring of ROS. *Circulation* **2003**, *108*, 1912–1916. [CrossRef]
31. Ebrahimian, T.; Li, M.W.; Lemarie, C.A.; Simeone, S.M.; Pagano, P.J.; Gaestel, M.; Paradis, P.; Wassmann, S.; Schiffrin, E.L. Mitogen-activated protein kinase-activated protein kinase 2 in angiotensin II-induced inflammation and hypertension: Regulation of oxidative stress. *Hypertension* **2011**, *57*, 245–254. [CrossRef] [PubMed]
32. Bedard, K.; Krause, K.H. The NOX family of ROS-generating NADPH oxidases: Physiology and pathophysiology. *Physiol. Rev.* **2007**, *87*, 245–313. [CrossRef] [PubMed]
33. Kobayashi, M.; Yamamoto, M. Molecular mechanisms activating the Nrf2-Keap1 pathway of antioxidant gene regulation. *Antioxid. Redox Signal.* **2005**, *7*, 385–394. [CrossRef] [PubMed]
34. Burke-Gaffney, A.; Evans, T.W. Lest we forget the endothelial glycocalyx in sepsis. *Crit. Care* **2012**, *16*, 121. [CrossRef] [PubMed]
35. Gumuz, M.P.; Kanmaz, B.; Buduneli, M. The role of oxidative stress in the interaction of periodontal disease with systemic diseases or conditions. *Oxid. Antioxid. Med. Sci.* **2016**, *5*, 33–38. [CrossRef]
36. Kinane, D.F.; Preshaw, P.M.; Loos, B.G. Working Group 2 of Seventh European Workshop on P. Host-response: Understanding the cellular and molecular mechanisms of host-microbial interactions—consensus of the Seventh European Workshop on Periodontology. *J. Clin. Periodontol.* **2011**, *38* (Suppl. S11), 44–48. [CrossRef] [PubMed]
37. Mousavi, S.; Bereswill, S.; Heimesaat, M.M. Immunomodulatory and Antimicrobial Effects of Vitamin C. *Eur. J. Microbiol. Immunol.* **2019**, *9*, 73–79. [CrossRef]

38. Carr, A.C.; Rosengrave, P.C.; Bayer, S.; Chambers, S.; Mehrtens, J.; Shaw, G.M. Hypovitaminosis C and vitamin C deficiency in critically ill patients despite recommended enteral and parenteral in takes. *Crit. Care* **2017**, *21*, 300. [CrossRef]
39. Carr, A.C.; Maggini, S. Vitamin C and Immune Function. *Nutrients* **2017**, *9*, 1211. [CrossRef]
40. Siti, H.N.; Kamisah, Y.; Kamsiah, J. The role of oxidative stress, antioxidants and vascular inflammation in cardiovascular disease (A review). *Vasc. Pharmacol.* **2015**, *71*, 40–56. [CrossRef]
41. Lykkesfeldt, J.; Tveden-Nyborg, P. The Pharmacokinetics of Vitamin C. *Nutrients* **2019**, *11*, 2412. [CrossRef] [PubMed]
42. Hemilä, H.; Chalker, E. Vitamin C Can Shorten the Length of Stay in the ICU: A Meta-Analysis. *Nutrients* **2019**, *11*, 708. [CrossRef] [PubMed]
43. Liugan, M.; Carr, A.C. Vitamin C and Neutrophil Function: Findings from Randomized Controlled Trials. *Nutrients* **2019**, *11*, 2102. [CrossRef] [PubMed]
44. Oudemans-van Straaten, H.M.; Spoelstra-de Man, A.M.; de Waard, M.C. Vitamin C revisited. *Crit. Care* **2014**, *18*, 460. [CrossRef]
45. Wang, Y.; Chun, O.K.; Song, W.O. Plasma and dietary antioxidant status as cardiovascular disease risk factors: A review of human studies. *Nutrients* **2013**, *5*, 2969–3004. [CrossRef]
46. Shaik-Dasthagirisaheb, Y.B.; Varvara, G.; Murmura, G.; Saggini, A.; Caraffa, A.; Antinolfi, P.; Tete, S.; Tripodi, D.; Conti, F.; Cianchetti, E.; et al. Role of vitamins D, E and C in immunity and inflammation. *J. Biol. Regul. Homeost. Agents* **2013**, *27*, 291–295.
47. Sailaja Devi, M.M.; Das, U.N. Effect of prostaglandins against alloxan-induced diabetes mellitus. *Prostaglandins Leukot. Essent. Fat. Acids* **2006**, *74*, 39–60. [CrossRef]
48. Das, U.N. Vitamin C for Type 2 Diabetes Mellitus and Hypertension. *Arch. Med Res.* **2019**, *50*, 11–14. [CrossRef]
49. Mason, S.A.; Rasmussen, B.; van Loon, L.J.C.; Salmon, J.; Wadley, G.D. Ascorbic acid supplementation improves postprandial glycaemic control and blood pressure in individuals with type 2 diabetes: Findings of a randomized cross-over trial. *Diabetes Obes. Metab.* **2019**, *21*, 674–682. [CrossRef]
50. Asmat, U.; Abad, K.; Ismail, K. Diabetes mellitus and oxidative stress-A concise review. *Saudi Pharm. J.* **2016**, *24*, 547–553. [CrossRef]
51. Maritim, A.C.; Sanders, R.A.; Watkins, J.B., 3rd. Diabetes, oxidative stress, and antioxidants: A review. *J. Biochem. Mol. Toxicol.* **2003**, *17*, 24–38. [CrossRef] [PubMed]
52. Erejuwa, O.O. Management of diabetes mellitus: Could simultaneous targeting of hyperglycemia and oxidative stress be a better panacea? *Int. J. Mol. Sci.* **2012**, *13*, 2965–2972. [CrossRef] [PubMed]
53. Nishida, M.; Grossi, S.G.; Dunford, R.G.; Ho, A.W.; Trevisan, M.; Genco, R.J. Dietary vitamin C and the risk for periodontal disease. *J. Periodontol.* **2000**, *71*, 1215–1223. [CrossRef] [PubMed]
54. Kuzmanova, D.; Jansen, I.D.; Schoenmaker, T.; Nazmi, K.; Teeuw, W.J.; Bizzarro, S.; Loos, B.G.; van der Velden, U. Vitamin C in plasma and leucocytes in relation to periodontitis. *J. Clin. Periodontol.* **2012**, *39*, 905–912. [CrossRef]
55. Petti, S.; Cairella, G.; Tarsitani, G. Nutritional variables related to gingival health in adolescent girls. *Community Dent. Oral Epidemiol.* **2000**, *28*, 407–413. [CrossRef]
56. Tada, A.; Miura, H. The Relationship between Vitamin C and Periodontal Diseases: A Systematic Review. *Int. J. Environ. Res. Public Health* **2019**, *16*, 2472. [CrossRef]
57. Monea, A.; Mezei, T.; Popsor, S.; Monea, M. Oxidative Stress: A Link between Diabetes Mellitus and Periodontal Disease. *Int. J. Endocrinol.* **2014**, *2014*, 917631. [CrossRef]
58. Li, X.; Sun, X.; Zhang, X.; Mao, Y.; Ji, Y.; Shi, L.; Cai, W.; Wang, P.; Wu, G.; Gan, X.; et al. Enhanced Oxidative Damage and Nrf2 Downregulation Contribute to the Aggravation of Periodontitis by Diabetes Mellitus. *Oxidative Med. Cell. Longev.* **2018**, *2018*, 9421019. [CrossRef]
59. Lee, J.H.; Shin, M.S.; Kim, E.J.; Ahn, Y.B.; Kim, H.D. The association of dietary vitamin C intake with periodontitis among Korean adults: Results from KNHANES. *PLoS ONE* **2017**, *12*, e0177074. [CrossRef]
60. Dietrich, T.; Kaye, E.K.; Nunn, M.E.; Van Dyke, T.; Garcia, R.I. Gingivitis susceptibility and its relation to periodontitis in men. *J. Dent. Res.* **2006**, *85*, 1134–1137. [CrossRef]
61. Isola, G.; Polizzi, A.; Muraglie, S.; Leonardi, R.; Lo Giudice, A. Assessment of Vitamin C and Antioxidant Profiles in Saliva and Serum in Patients with Periodontitis and Ischemic Heart Disease. *Nutrients* **2019**, *11*, 2956. [CrossRef] [PubMed]

62. Moher, D.; Liberati, A.; Tetzlaff, J.; Altman, D.G.; PRISMA Group. Preferred reporting items for systematic reviews and meta-analyses: The PRISMA statement. *PLoS Med.* **2009**, *6*, e1000097. [CrossRef] [PubMed]
63. Gokhale, N.H.; Acharya, A.B.; Patil, V.S.; Trivedi, D.J.; Thakur, S.L. A Short-Term Evaluation of the Relationship Between Plasma Ascorbic Acid Levels and Periodontal Disease in Systemically Healthy and Type 2 Diabetes Mellitus Subjects. *J. Diet. Suppl.* **2013**, *10*, 93–104. [CrossRef] [PubMed]
64. Kunsongkeit, P.; Okuma, N.; Rassameemasmaung, S.; Chaivanit, P. Effect of vitamin C as an adjunct in nonsurgical periodontal therapy in uncontrolled type 2 diabetes mellitus patients. *Eur. J. Dent.* **2019**, *13*, 444–449. [CrossRef]
65. Thomas, B.; Kumari, S.; Ramitha, K.; Ashwini Kumari, M.B. Ashwini Kumari, Comparative evaluation of micronutrient status in the serum of diabetes mellitus patients and healthy individuals with periodontitis. *J. Indian Soc. Periodontol.* **2010**, *14*, 46–49. [CrossRef]
66. Gümüş, P.; Buduneli, N.; Cetinkalp, S.; Hawkins, S.I.; Renaud, D.; Kinane, D.F.; Scott, D.A. Salivary antioxidants in patients with type 1 or 2 diabetes and inflammatory periodontal disease: A case-control study. *J. Periodontol.* **2009**, *80*, 1440–1446. [CrossRef]
67. Patil, V.S.; Patil, V.P.; Gokhale, N.; Acharya, A.; Kangokar, P. Chronic periodontitis in type 2 diabetes mellitus: Oxidative stress as a common factor in periodontal tissue injury. *J. Clin. Diagn. Res.* **2016**, *10*, 12–16. [CrossRef]
68. Amaliya, A.; Laine, M.L.; Delanghe, J.R.; Loos, B.G.; Van Wijk, A.J.; Van der Velden, U. Javaproject on periodontal diseases. Periodontal bone loss in relation to environmental to environmental and systemic conditions. *J. Clin. Periodontol.* **2015**, *42*, 325–332. [CrossRef]
69. Bogdan, M.; Silosi, I.; Surlin, P.; Tica, A.A.; Tica, O.S.; Balseanu, T.A.; Rauten, A.M.; Camen, A. Salivary and serum biomarkers for the study of side effects of aripiprazole coprescribed with mirtazapine in rats. *Int. J. Clin. Exp. Med.* **2015**, *8*, 8051–8059.
70. Gariballa, S. Poor vitamin C status is associated with increased depression symptoms following acute illness in older people. *Int. J. Vitam. Nutr Res.* **2014**, *84*, 12–17. [CrossRef]
71. Kocot, J.; Luchowska-Kocot, D.; Kielczykowska, M.; Musik, I.; Kurzepa, J. Does Vitamin C Influence Neurodegenerative Diseases and Psychiatric Disorders? *Nutrients* **2017**, *9*, 659. [CrossRef] [PubMed]
72. Salinero-Fort, M.A.; Gómez-Campelo, P.; San Andrés-Rebollo, F.J.; Cárdenas-Valladolid, J.; Abánades-Herranz, J.C.; Carrillo de Santa Pau, E.; Chico-Moraleja, R.M.; Beamud-Victoria, D.; de Miguel-Yanes, J.M.; Jimenez-Garcia, R.; et al. Prevalence of depression in patients with type 2 diabetes mellitus in Spain (the DIADEMA Study): Results from the MADIABETES cohort. *BMJ Open* **2018**, *8*, e020768. [CrossRef] [PubMed]
73. Hwang, S.H.; Park, S.G. The relationship between depression and periodontal diseases. *Community Dent. Health* **2018**, *35*, 23–29. [PubMed]
74. Ward, M.S.; Lamb, J.; May, J.M.; Harrison, F.E. Behavioral and monoamine changes following severe vitamin C deficiency. *J. Neurochem.* **2013**, *124*, 363–375. [CrossRef]
75. Moretti, M.; Colla, A.; de Oliveira Balen, G.; dos Santos, D.B.; Budni, J.; de Freitas, A.E.; Farina, M.; Severo Rodrigues, A.L. Ascorbic acid treatment, similarly to fluoxetine, reverses depressive-like behavior and brain oxidative damage induced by chronic unpredictable stress. *J. Psychiatr. Res.* **2012**, *46*, 331–340. [CrossRef]
76. Badescu, S.V.; Tataru, C.; Kobylinska, L.; Georgescu, E.L.; Zahiu, D.M.; Zagrean, A.M.; Zagrean, L. The association between Diabetes mellitus and Depression. *J. Med. Life* **2016**, *9*, 120–125.
77. Fatima, Z.; Bey, A.; Azmi, S.A.; Gupta, N.D.; Khan, A. Mental depression as a risk factor for periodontal disease: A case-control study. *Gen. Dent.* **2016**, *5*, 86–89. [CrossRef]
78. Penmetsa, G.S.; Seethalakshmi, P. Effect of stress, depression, and anxiety over periodontal health indicators among health professional students. *J. Indian Assoc. Public Health Dent.* **2019**, *17*, 36–40.
79. Nascimento, G.G.; Gastal, M.T.; Leite, F.R.M.; Quevedo, L.A.; Peres, K.G.; Peres, M.A.; Horta, B.L.; Barros, F.C.; Demarco, F.F. Is there an association between depression and periodontitis? A birth cohort study. *J. Clin. Periodontol.* **2019**, *46*, 31–39. [CrossRef]
80. Turcu-Stiolica, A.; Taerel, A.E.; Turcu-Stiolica, R. Identifying and measuring compliance and adherence in antidepressants taking. *Procedia Econ. Financ.* **2014**, *15*, 836–839. [CrossRef]
81. Kroenke, K.; Spitzer, R.L.; Williams, J.B.; Lowe, B. The Patient Health Questionnaire Somatic, Anxiety, and Depressive Symptom Scales: A systematic review. *Gen. Hosp. Psychiatry* **2010**, *32*, 345–359. [CrossRef] [PubMed]

82. Kaur, G.; Kathariya, R.; Bansal, S.; Singh, A.; Shahakar, D. Dietary antioxidants and their indispensable role in periodontal health. *J. Food Drug Anal.* **2016**, *24*, 239–246. [CrossRef] [PubMed]
83. Muniz, F.W.; Nogueira, S.B.; Mendes, F.L.; Rösing, C.K.; Moreira, M.M.; de Andrade, G.M.; Carvalho Rde, S. The impact of antioxidant agents complimentary to periodontal therapy on oxidative stress and periodontal outcomes: A systematic review. *Arch. Oral Biol.* **2015**, *60*, 1203–1214. [CrossRef] [PubMed]

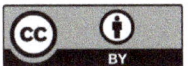

© 2020 by the authors. Licensee MDPI, Basel, Switzerland. This article is an open access article distributed under the terms and conditions of the Creative Commons Attribution (CC BY) license (http://creativecommons.org/licenses/by/4.0/).

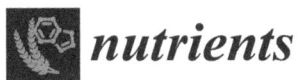

Review

Do Dietary Supplements and Nutraceuticals Have Effects on Dental Implant Osseointegration? A Scoping Review

Livia Nastri [1], Antimo Moretti [1,*], Silvia Migliaccio [2], Marco Paoletta [1], Marco Annunziata [1], Sara Liguori [1], Giuseppe Toro [1], Massimiliano Bianco [1], Gennaro Cecoro [1], Luigi Guida [1] and Giovanni Iolascon [1]

1. Department of Medical and Surgical Specialties and Dentistry, University of Campania "Luigi Vanvitelli", 80138 Naples, Italy; livia.nastri@unicampania.it (L.N.); paolettamarco@libero.it (M.P.); marco.annunziata@unicampania.it (M.A.); s.liguori@hotmail.it (S.L.); peppetoro@msn.com (G.T.); massimiliano.bianco27@gmail.com (M.B.); gennarocecoro@gmail.com (G.C.); luigi.guida@unicampania.it (L.G.); giovanni.iolascon@gmail.com (G.I.)
2. Department of Movement, Human and Health Sciences, Unit Endocrinology, University Foro Italico, 00135 Rome, Italy; silvia.migliaccio@uniroma4.it
* Correspondence: antimomor83@hotmail.it; Tel.: +39-08-1566-5537

Received: 27 December 2019; Accepted: 18 January 2020; Published: 20 January 2020

Abstract: Several factors affect dental implant osseointegration, including surgical issues, bone quality and quantity, and host-related factors, such as patients' nutritional status. Many micronutrients might play a key role in dental implant osseointegration by influencing some alveolar bone parameters, such as healing of the alveolus after tooth extraction. This scoping review aims to summarize the role of dietary supplements in optimizing osseointegration after implant insertion surgery. A technical expert panel (TEP) of 11 medical specialists with expertise in oral surgery, bone metabolism, nutrition, and orthopedic surgery performed the review following the PRISMA-ScR (Preferred Reporting Items for Systematic Reviews and Meta-Analyses Extension for Scoping Reviews) model. The TEP identified micronutrients from the "European Union (EU) Register of nutrition and health claims made on foods" that have a relationship with bone and tooth health, and planned a PubMed search, selecting micronutrients previously identified as MeSH (Medical Subject Headings) terms and adding to each of them the words "dental implants" and "osseointegration". The TEP identified 19 studies concerning vitamin D, magnesium, resveratrol, vitamin C, a mixture of calcium, magnesium, zinc, and vitamin D, and synthetic bone mineral. However, several micronutrients are non-authorized by the "EU Register on nutrition and health claims" for improving bone and/or tooth health. Our scoping review suggests a limited role of nutraceuticals in promoting osseointegration of dental implants, although, in some cases, such as for vitamin D deficiency, there is a clear link among their deficit, reduced osseointegration, and early implant failure, thus requiring an adequate supplementation.

Keywords: dietary supplements; dental implants; osseointegration; vitamin D; magnesium; resveratrol; ascorbic acid; zinc; calcium; bone

1. Introduction

Osseointegration is defined as "a process whereby a clinically asymptomatic rigid fixation of alloplastic materials is achieved and maintained in bone during functional loading" [1]. Osseointegration is involved in dental implants healing, thus leading to a functional unit that may rehabilitate one or more missing teeth, supporting dental prosthesis.

In addition to key factors that affect the osseointegration, such as the surgical technique, bone quality and quantity, postoperative inflammation or infection, smoking habits, and implant material and surface [2–7], other factors should be taken into account, including the immunological and nutritional status of the host. Alongside the promotion of a healthy diet, such as the Mediterranean one, to achieve a desirable general health status, recently, increasing attention was paid to promoting the consumption of micronutrients that could have benefits on health and resistance to diseases [8].

Several micronutrients affecting bone metabolism were demonstrated to have an influence on skeletal system; in particular, calcium, fluorides, magnesium, potassium, vitamin B6, vitamin D, and zinc positively influence bone health, reducing the risk of fracture [9]. In addition, fat-, carbohydrate-, and cholesterol-rich diets and reduced calcium intake exhibit detrimental influences on jaw bone and alveolar bone [10]. Therefore, a specific diet regimen and micronutrients might play a key role in the different phases of dental implant osseointegration.

Recent evidence demonstrated that some nutritional regimens directly influence alveolar bone parameters in experimental models of periodontitis [11–13], orthodontic tooth movement [14], and bone repair after tooth extraction [15]. In particular, it was demonstrated that diet (in its different meanings of macro- and micronutrients) can affect the healing of the alveolus after tooth extraction, influencing both the morphology and the quality of alveolar bone [15].

Bone tissue repair mechanisms and bone metabolism are strongly influenced by nutritional aspects and are crucial to obtaining proper bone restoration optimizing osseointegration processes.

The aim of this scoping review is to summarize the state of the art regarding the role of micronutrients, currently available in nutraceuticals or dietary supplements, on dental implantology, highlighting which of them, supported by evidence-based medicine (EBM), might effectively have an influence on the achievement and the maintenance of osseointegration after implant insertion surgery.

2. Materials and Methods

In performing this scoping review, we followed the PRISMA-ScR (Preferred Reporting Items for Systematic Reviews and Meta-Analyses Extension for Scoping Reviews) model [16].

As a first step, a technical expert panel (TEP) consisting of 11 medical specialists was established. In particular, the TEP was composed of two oral surgeons with expertise in osseointegrated dental implants, two periodontists with expertise in peri-implant oral tissues physiology and pathology, three bone specialists, two experts on scoping review methodology, one nutritionist, and one orthopedic surgeon.

2.1. Search Strategy

The TEP selected micronutrients from the "European Union (EU) Register of nutrition and health claims made on foods" that have a relationship with bone and tooth health, included in dietary supplements and nutraceuticals. Therefore, the TEP planned a research on PubMed (Public MedLine, run by the National Center of Biotechnology Information, NCBI, of the National Library of Medicine of Bethesda, Bethesda, MD, USA), selecting micronutrients as MeSH (Medical Subject Headings) terms; to each of them, the following terms were added to run the PubMed Search Builder: "dental implants", "osseointegration". For example: ("Vitamin D" [Mesh]) AND "Dental Implants" [Mesh]) (see Supplementary Materials, Table S1).

2.2. Study Selection

According to the objective of the study, the TEP defined the characteristics of the sources of evidence, considering for eligibility any researches published in medical literature in the last 10 years (last update on 16 October 2019), including only those in the English language.

2.3. Data Extraction and Quality Assessment

All types of studies were included in our scoping review, both pre-clinical (in vitro and animal studies) and clinical studies. Methodological quality assessment was made according to the EBM pyramid: meta-analysis, systematic review, randomized controlled trial (RCT), cohort study, case–control study, case series, and case report.

Finally, the TEP summarized the resulting micronutrients with effective and safe daily doses that improve bone and tooth health.

3. Results

From the micronutrients listed in the "EU Register of nutrition and health claims made on foods", the TEP selected the following 18 nutraceuticals that may have influence on bone and teeth: calcium, fluorides, magnesium, potassium, resveratrol, vitamin C (ascorbic acid), vitamin D, vitamin E (alpha-tocopherol), vitamin K2 (menaquinone-7, MK7), zinc, vitamin A, vitamin B1 (thiamine), vitamin B2 (riboflavin), vitamin B3 (niacinamide), vitamin B5 (pantothenic acid), vitamin B6, vitamin B7 (biotin), and vitamin B12 (Table 1). However, according to the "EU Register of nutrition and health claims made on foods", fluoride is non-authorized for supporting bone mineralization, and potassium is non-authorized for maintaining tooth mineralization, whereas vitamin B2, vitamin E, vitamin A, vitamin B1, vitamin B2, vitamin B3, vitamin B6, vitamin B7, and vitamin B12 are non-authorized for both functions. Moreover, potassium and zinc are not considered to influence tooth metabolism, while vitamin K2, resveratrol, and vitamin B5 are not recommended for bone and tooth metabolism according to the "EU Register of nutrition and health claims made on foods". Among these substances, we found studies concerning nutraceuticals and dental implants or osseointegration only for vitamin D, magnesium, resveratrol, vitamin C, a mixture of calcium, magnesium, zinc, and vitamin D, and synthetic bone mineral (a supplement containing calcium, phosphate, magnesium, zinc, fluoride, and carbonate).

Table 1. Effects of selected micronutrients on bone and tooth health.

Nutrient or Non-Nutrient Compound	Effect
Calcium	99% of calcium in the body is in the form of hydroxyapatite, which is bone and tooth mineral [17]. Relationship between calcium and maintenance of normal bone and tooth assessed with a favorable outcome (European Food Safety Authority (EFSA) opinion).
Fluorides	Stimulates osteoblast growth and bone formation, increasing bone mineral density (BMD) [18], and supports tooth mineralization (EFSA opinion).
Magnesium	Essential for the conversion of vitamin D into its active form and necessary for calcium absorption and metabolism [19], and maintenance of normal bone and teeth (EFSA opinion).
Potassium	Potassium citrate helps maintain acid–base balance and support bone health, counteracting bone resorption [20]. However, a cause-and-effect relationship is not established between the dietary intake of potassium salts of citric acid and maintenance of normal bone (EFSA opinion).
Resveratrol	Active substance found in food, such as red grapes, peanuts, and berries, with anti-inflammatory and antioxidant effects; it additionally provides an inhibitory effect on osteoclast differentiation and potentially induces bone formation [21] (EFSA opinion about bone and tooth health not available).
Vitamin C (ascorbic acid)	Enhances osteoblastogenesis and inhibits osteoclastogenesis via Wnt/β-catenin signaling [22]. Vitamin C contributes to normal function of bones and teeth (EFSA opinion).
Vitamin D	Modulates calcium and phosphate metabolism; it promotes growth, bone mineralization of the skeleton and teeth [17], and maintenance of normal bone and teeth (EFSA opinion).

Table 1. *Cont.*

Nutrient or Non-Nutrient Compound	Effect
Vitamin E (alpha-tocopherol)	Reduces the expression of receptor activator of nuclear factor kappa B (NF-κB) ligand (RANKL) in osteoblasts and inhibits osteoclastogenesis [23]. However, a cause-and-effect relationship is not established between the dietary intake of vitamin E and maintenance of normal bone and teeth (EFSA opinion).
Vitamin K2 (MK7)	Stimulates osteoblasts differentiation, protects these cells from apoptosis [24], and maintains normal bone (EFSA opinion).
Zinc	Stimulates osteoblast proliferation, differentiation, and mineralization, which may facilitate bone formation [25,26] and maintain normal bone (EFSA opinion).
Vitamin A	Increases the effect of bone morphogenetic proteins (BMPs) on osteogenic differentiation [27]. A cause-and-effect relationship is not established between the dietary intake of vitamin A and maintenance of normal bone and teeth (EFSA opinion).
B Vitamins	Deficiency in folic acid and vitamins B6 and B12 can result in increased serum homocysteine that leads to endothelial dysfunction (decreased bone blood flow) and enhanced osteoclast activity (bone resorption). Moreover, hyperhomocysteinemia interferes with cross-linking of collagen (altered bone matrix) [28]. However, a cause-and-effect relationship is not established between the dietary intake of B vitamins and maintenance of normal bone and teeth (EFSA opinion).

In particular, we included 11 studies concerning vitamin D, of which five were clinical studies (three retrospective studies, one case series, and one case report), and six were preclinical studies on animals: two preclinical studies on animals concerning magnesium, two preclinical studies on animals for resveratrol, one preclinical study on animals concerning the supplementation with a combination of calcium, magnesium, zinc and vitamin D, two preclinical studies on animals concerning synthetic bone mineral (composed by dicalcium phosphate dihydrate and magnesium and zinc chlorides), and one clinical study concerning vitamin C supplementation (Figure 1, Table 2).

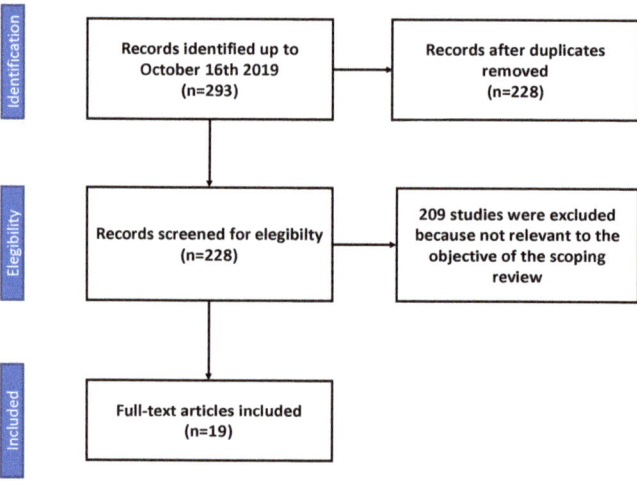

Figure 1. Flow diagram of sources selection process.

Table 2. Relevant data from each study included in the scoping review.

Author, Year	Nutraceutical Compound	Study Design/Experimental Model	Main Aim	Results
Mangano et al., 2018 [29]	Vitamin D	Retrospective study	To investigate the correlation between serum levels of vitamin D and early dental implant failure	In patients with serum levels of vitamin D < 10 ng/mL, there were 11.1% early dental implant failures (EDIF; failures that occurred before prosthesis positioning), 4.4% EDIFs in patients with vitamin D levels between 10 and 30 ng/mL, and 2.9% EDIFs in patients with levels > 30 ng/mL. No statistically significant correlation was found between EDIF and vitamin D serum levels, but a clear trend toward an increased incidence of EDIF with lowering of serum vitamin D levels was reported.
Wagner et al., 2017 [30]	Vitamin D	Retrospective parallel group	To evaluate the influence of osteoporosis on the marginal peri-implant bone level	Osteoporosis was shown to have a significant negative influence on the marginal bone loss (MBL) at the mesial and the distal implant aspect. Vitamin D positively and significantly affected the MBL, showing beneficial effects on the peri-implant bone formation.
Mangano et al., 2016 [31]	Vitamin D	Retrospective study	To investigate the correlation between early dental implant failure and low serum levels of vitamin D	There were 9% EDIFs in patients with serum levels of vitamin D < 10 ng/mL, 3.9% EDIFs in patients with vitamin D levels between 10 and 30 ng/mL, and 2.2% EDIFs in patients with vitamin D levels > 30 ng/mL. Although there was an increasing trend in the incidence of early implant failures with the worsening of vitamin D deficiency, the difference between these 3 groups was not statistically significant.
Fretwurst et al., 2016 [32]	Vitamin D	Case series	To evaluate the correlation between vitamin D deficiency and early implant failure	After vitamin D supplementation, implant placement was successful in 2 patients with previous early implant failures.
Bryce & Macbeth, 2014 [33]	Vitamin D	Case report	To investigate the influence of vitamin D deficiency in the osseointegration process of a dental implant	Authors reported a case of a patient that received dental extraction and the insertion of an immediate implant that failed to osseointegrate. Medical investigations revealed that he was severely vitamin D-deficient and that this may have contributed to the implant failure.
Liu et al., 2014 [34]	Vitamin D	Animal study	To investigate the effect of Vitamin D supplementation on implant osseointegration in CKD mice.	In rats with chronic kidney disease (CKD), vitamin D supplementation led to bone-to-implant contact rate (BIC) and bone volume/total volume levels higher than the CKD group without supplementation and comparable to rats without CKD. Also, at the push-in test, the CKD + vitamin D group had better results than the CKD group, which were comparable to the control group.

Table 2. Cont.

Author, Year	Nutraceutical Compound	Study Design/Experimental Model	Main Aim	Results
Zhou et al., 2012 [35]	Vitamin D	Animal study	Investigate the effects of 1,25(OH)2D3 on implant osseointegration in osteoporotic rats	Vitamin D supplementation in osteoporotic rats led to formation of more cancellous bone around implants, an increase of bone volume by 96.0% in terms of osseointegration, by 94.4% in terms of mean trabecular number, by 112.5% in terms of mean trabecular thickness, by 51.8% in terms of trabecular connective density, and by 38.0% in terms of connective density, as well as a decrease in terms of trabecular separation by 39.3%. Vitamin D increased bone area density by 1.2-fold and bone-to-implant contact by 1.5-fold and increased the maximal push-out force by 2.0-fold.
Wu et al., 2012 [36]	Vitamin D	Animal study	Effect of insulin and vitamin D3 on implant osseointegration in diabetic mellitus rats	Vitamin D and insulin combined treatment of diabetic rats led to an improvement of bone volume per total volume, percentage of osseointegration, mean trabecular thickness, mean trabecular number, connective density, maximal push-out force, and ultimate shear strength, BIC, and bone area ratio (BA), while the mean trabecular separation decreased. These indexes showed values comparable to those of healthy control rats.
Akhavan et al., 2012 [37]	Vitamin D	Animal study	Compare the effect of vitamin D administration on bone to implant contact in diabetic rats	At the histological analysis 3 weeks after implant insertion, diabetic rats reported a BIC level of 44 ± 19, while diabetic rats receiving vitamin D had a level of 57 ± 20. At 6 weeks, the control group reported BIC level of 70 ± 29 and the vitamin D group had a level of 65 ± 22. Considering these results, vitamin D seems not to have an effect on osseointegration of implants in diabetic rats.
Dvorak et al., 2012 [38]	Vitamin D (deficiency)	Animal study	Impact of vitamin D supplementation on the process of osseointegration	Vitamin D depletion in ovariectomized rats led to a significant decrease in bone-to-implant contact in the cortical area compared to rats fed with a standard vitamin D diet, while no significant reduction in BIC was observed in the medullar and the periosteal compartment.
Kelly et al., 2008 [39]	Vitamin D (deficiency)	Animal study	To evaluate the effect of a common deficiency of vitamin D on implant osseointegration in the rat model	Vitamin D deficiency in rats, 14 days after implant insertion, led to a lower push-in test and a lower BIC, compared to rats without deficiency. SEM analyses showed that the calcified tissues after push-in test, in the vitamin D deficiency groups, fractured between the implant and the surrounding tissue, resulting in exposed implant surface.

Table 2. Cont.

Author, Year	Nutraceutical Compound	Study Design/Experimental Model	Main Aim	Results
Belluci et al., 2011 [40]	Magnesium	Animal study	To evaluate the effect of magnesium dietary deficiency on bone metabolism and bone tissue around implants with established osseointegration	Rats fed with a diet with 90% magnesium reduction presented loss of systemic bone mass, decreased cortical bone thickness, and lower values of removal torque of the implants.
Del Barrio et al., 2010 [41]	Magnesium	Animal study	To evaluate the effect of severe magnesium dietary deficiency on systemic bone density and biomechanical resistance of bone tissue to the removal torque of osseointegrated implants	Magnesium intake reduction of 90% in diet of rats led to a statistically lower removal torque of the implants compared to rats fed with the recommended magnesium content, while no difference was demonstrated between the group with a 75% magnesium reduction and the control group.
Ribeiro et al., 2018 [42]	Resveratrol	Animal study	To investigate the effect of resveratrol on peri-implant repair, and its influence on bone-related markers in rats	Systemic assumption of resveratrol positively affected biomechanical retention of titanium implants, measured as torque removal values, and determined a higher BIC in smoking rats, when compared to smoking + placebo rat group.
Casarin et al., 2014 [43]	Resveratrol	Animal study	To investigate the effect of resveratrol on bone healing and its influence on the gene expression of osteogenic markers	Resveratrol increased the counter-torque values of implant removal when compared to placebo therapy and increased bone healing of critical size defects in rats.
Pimentel et al., 2016 [44]	Calcium, magnesium, zinc, and vitamin D3	Animal study	To investigate the effect of micronutrients supplementation on the bone repair around implants	Rats receiving calcium, magnesium, zinc, and vitamin D intake for 30 days after implant insertion showed counter-torque values with no statistical difference compared to rats that received a placebo solution. Neither bone volume per total volume nor BIC showed a statistically significant difference between the 2 groups.

Table 2. Cont.

Author, Year	Nutraceutical Compound	Study Design/Experimental Model	Main Aim	Results
Takahashi et al., 2016 [45]	Synthetic bone mineral (dicalcium phosphate dihydrate + magnesium and zinc chlorides)	Animal study	To investigate whether oral intake of synthetic bone mineral improves peri-implant bone formation and bone micro architecture	Synthetic bone mineral (SBM; a mixture of dicalcium phosphate dihydrate and magnesium and zinc chlorides) intake led to a significantly higher bone volume per total volume, trabecular thickness, trabecular star volume compared to rats fed without SBM. The bone surface ratio of the rats that were fed with SBM was significantly lower than that of the rats fed without SBM. The trabecular number of the rats fed with SBM was not significantly increased compared to rats fed without SBM. Rats fed without SBM had no bone formation at 2 weeks, while bone formation was clearly observed in rats fed with SBM at 2 and 4 weeks after implantation. In rats fed without SBM at 4 weeks after implantation, irregular bone bands around the implants were observed.
Watanabe et al., 2015 [46]	Synthetic bone mineral (dicalcium phosphate dihydrate + magnesium and zinc chlorides)	Animal study	To investigate the effect of synthetic bone mineral in accelerating peri-implant bone formation	Pull-out strength was greatly higher in the SBM group compared to control group at 2 and 4 weeks. Bone mineral density was approximately double in the SBM group compared to control group both at 2 and 4 weeks, and this result was confirmed also by bone mineral density (BMD) color imaging. Microscopy observation showed green fluorescence in the SBM group at 2 and 4 weeks and only at 4 weeks in the control group.
Li et al., 2018 [47]	Vitamin C	Parallel group	To explore the effects of vitamin C supplementation in wound healing, following the placement of dental implants with or without bone grafts and patients with chronic periodontitis	Patients that received implants with guided bone regeneration (GBR) or with Bio-Oss collagen grafts and received vitamin C supplements, 14 days post-surgery, showed significantly improved wound healing compared with patients receiving the same surgical therapy but without vitamin C supplements. Patients suffering from chronic periodontitis that received implants showed significantly better wound healing at 7 and 14 days when they had vitamin C supplements compared to patients without supplements. Vitamin C showed no postoperative pain relief proprieties in any group.

3.1. Vitamin D

3.1.1. Animal Studies

In our scoping review, we included six preclinical studies on animal models, more precisely, on rats.

Liu et al., in 2014 [34], found that vitamin D supplementation in rats affected by chronic kidney disease (CKD) improved bone-to-implant contact (BIC) compared to CKD rats that did not receive vitamin D, making this finding comparable to that of rats without CKD. Also, the bone volume in the circumferential zone within 100 mm of the implant surface increased after vitamin D administration. At two weeks, the push-in test showed significantly better results for the vitamin D-treated group compared to untreated CKD mice.

Zhou et al., in 2012 [35], demonstrated that vitamin D supplementation in osteoporotic rats, eight weeks after implantation, improved bone volume, osseointegration, mean trabecular number, mean trabecular thickness, and trabecular connective density, while it decreased trabecular separation, as well as increased bone area density, BIC, and the maximal push-out force.

Wu et al., in 2012 [36], inserted titanium implants in diabetic rats and evaluated the effects of different kinds of diabetes therapies. The combined therapy with insulin and vitamin D showed the best effects on osseointegration, bone volume, mean trabecular thickness, mean trabecular number, connective density, mean trabecular separation, push out force, shear strength, BIC, and bone area ratio. Treatments with vitamin D or insulin only showed better results compared to untreated diabetic rats, but worse than the combined therapy. All the parameters listed above, in the combined treatment group, resulted similar to those of the control healthy group.

Akhavan et al., in 2012 [37], evaluated the effects of vitamin D supplementation on BIC in diabetic rats compared to a placebo group. At three weeks, the vitamin D group showed higher values of BIC compared to the placebo group, and also at six weeks, even if in a non-statistically significant way, leading the authors to conclude that vitamin D seems to not have an effect on the osseointegration of implants in diabetic rats.

Dvorak et al., in 2012 [38], showed that, in osteoporotic rats, a vitamin D depletion led to a significant decrease in BIC in the cortical area. In rats that received a vitamin D-free diet, followed by vitamin D repletion, no significant difference could be found compared to the control group that received a standard vitamin D diet.

Kelly et al., in 2008 [39], found that vitamin D deficiency, 14 days after implantation, led to a lower push-in test and a decreased BIC compared to a normal vitamin D status.

3.1.2. Clinical Studies

The clinical studies on vitamin D that we included in this scoping review were three retrospective studies, one case series, and one case report.

From the retrospective studies of Mangano et al. of 2016 [31] and 2018 [29], it emerged that, in patients with vitamin D deficiency, there were a higher percentage of early dental implant failures (failures that occurred before prosthesis positioning, EDIF). However, although there was a clear trend toward an increased incidence of EDIF with lower serum 25(OH)D, no statistically significant difference was found among the three groups with different vitamin D status.

In the retrospective study of Wagner et al. of 2017 [30], osteoporosis was shown to have a significant negative influence on marginal bone loss around implants, but vitamin D significantly affected the marginal bone loss at the mesial and distal implant aspect, showing beneficial effects on the peri-implant bone formation.

Fretwurst et al., in 2016 [32], reported two cases of implant failures occurring within 15 days of surgery in patients with vitamin D deficiency; in one patient, there were even two consecutive implant failures. In both patients, after vitamin D supplementation, implants were placed successfully. The authors also noticed that failures were sometimes associated with pain and discomfort in vitamin D-deficient patients.

Also, Bryce and Macbeth, in 2014 [33], reported a case of missed osseointegration in a patient affected by severe vitamin D deficiency.

3.1.3. Magnesium

We included two animal studies that evaluated the effects of magnesium deficiency on osseointegration of titanium implants. The deficiency of magnesium led to lower cortical bone thickness, lower values of removal torque of the implants, and lower bone mineral density (BMD) [40,41]. In detail,

Bellucci et al., in 2011 [40], found that a 90% reduction of magnesium intake, 90 days after implant insertion, led to lower BMD values. In the magnesium reduction group, upper and lower cortical thicknesses were significantly reduced, as well as the removal torque of the implants. On the other hand, the radiographic bone density and cortical thickness around the implants resulted similar between the two groups.

Del Barrio et al., in 2010 [41], reported that only a 90% reduced magnesium intake resulted in low BMD after implant insertion compared to both a 75% magnesium intake reduction and a normal magnesium intake.

3.1.4. Resveratrol

We found two animal studies that evaluated the effects of resveratrol intake on the osseointegration of titanium implants.

In 2018, Ribeiro et al. [42] demonstrated that supplementation of resveratrol led to an improvement in counter-torque and BIC in rats exposed to cigarette smoking, compared to rats exposed to cigarette smoking but receiving placebo. This finding seems quite relevant, considering that detrimental effects of smoking on oral health in terms of increased postoperative infections and marginal bone loss in patients receiving dental implants are well established [48–50]. Also, Casarin et al., in 2014 [43], demonstrated that resveratrol intake had positive effects on the biomechanical retention of the implants, because there were significantly higher average counter-torque values for implant removal in rats that received resveratrol.

3.1.5. Mixtures of Micronutrients

Pimentel et al., in 2016 [44], evaluated the effects of a mixture of calcium, magnesium, zinc, and vitamin D on rats that received titanium implants. They found that there was no statistically significant difference among the counter-torque values for implant removal, bone volume, and BIC in the placebo group when compared to the micronutrient group.

Takahashi et al., in 2016 [45], evaluated the effects of supplementation with synthetic bone mineral (SBM), a mixture of calcium phosphate dihydrate and magnesium and zinc chlorides, on titanium implants in osteoporotic rats. They found significantly higher bone volume and lower bone surface ratio in the SBM group. Moreover, the trabecular thickness increased significantly from two to four weeks after implant insertion in treated group, while the improvement of the same parameters was not significant in the control group. Also, other histomorphometric parameters significantly improved in SBM group, such as the trabecular star volume, although the between-group difference in terms of trabecular number was not significant. Finally, rats receiving SBM showed enhanced bone formation, evaluated by micro-computed tomography (micro-CT), both at two and at four weeks compared to rats fed without SBM.

Also, Watanabe et al., in 2015 [46], evaluated the effects of SBM on osseointegration in rats. They found that pull-out strength in the treated group was six times higher than in the control group two weeks after implantation and twice higher at four weeks. The BMD in the SBM group was approximately double compared to the control group at two weeks and more than double at four weeks. BMD color imaging showed that the control group colors mainly ranged from blue to yellow at two and four weeks after implantation, while the SBM group mainly occupied the orange and red end of the spectrum at two and four weeks after implantation. Given that blue and light blue, green and yellow, and orange and red represent low, medium, and high BMD, respectively, the BMD color imaging indicated that peri-implant bone had a higher BMD in the SBM group than in the control group. Fluorescence microscopy imaging of the control group revealed no green fluorescence at two weeks after implantation. However, green fluorescence was clearly observed in the SBM group at two and four weeks after implantation, while irregular bands appeared around the implants in the control group at four weeks.

3.2. Vitamin C

Li et al., in 2018 [47], evaluated the effects of vitamin C supplementation on four populations: patients receiving dental implants by guided bone regeneration (GBR), patients treated with Bio-Oss collagen, patients with chronic periodontitis receiving dental implants, and a control group without any bone grafting or periodontal disease. The authors found that vitamin C supplementation improved postoperative wound healing following dental implant surgery in patients with chronic periodontitis and in those treated with GBR or Bio-Oss collagen grafts. However, vitamin C supplementation was ineffective in decreasing the postoperative pain associated with dental implant surgery.

4. Discussion

To the best of our knowledge, this is the first scoping review to investigate the putative role of dietary supplements in affecting bone structural and mechanical properties involved in dental implant osseointegration, as well as in improving clinical outcomes, such as the maintenance of peri-implant tissue health and implant success rate.

The Federal Food, Drug, and Cosmetic Act defines a dietary supplement as a product that is intended to supplement the diet, which bears or contains one or more ingredients including a vitamin, mineral, herb, and amino acid, or a concentrate, metabolite, constituent, extract, or combinations of these [50]. The term "nutraceutical" was coined by Stephen De Felice to define "food (or parts of a food) that provides medical or health benefits, including the prevention and/or treatment of a disease", by the fusion of the words "nutrition" and "pharmaceutical", commonly used in marketing with no regulatory legal definition [51]. Ten years later, nutraceuticals are defined as dietary supplements that include a concentrated form of a presumed bioactive substance, originally derived from a food, but present in a non-food matrix, and used to maintain or improve health status in dosages exceeding those obtainable from conventional foods [52].

It should be stressed, however, that there is no consensus with regard to "nutraceutical" definition or similar terms. Aronson recently considered that the term "nutraceuticals" is too vague and should be abandoned, even if he did not propose any robust alternatives [53].

According to the recent data of the United States (US) Centers for Disease Control and Prevention's National Health and Nutrition Examination Survey (NHANES), more than 25% of the US population had an insufficient intake of vitamins A, C, D, and E, as well as calcium, magnesium, and potassium in their diet; thus, the modern diet of Western countries does not seem to have an adequate intake of micronutrients. It was reported that micronutrient deficiencies affect around two billion people worldwide [54]. However, a consensus about the use of these substances, particularly concerning the adequate amount and safety, is not yet reached, even if they are supposed to have multiple physiological beneficial effects.

Several micronutrients are hypothesized to have an influence on skeletal system, particularly on jaw bone and alveolar bone [9] and on dental implant osseointegration. However, according to our findings, very few elements (i.e., vitamin D, magnesium, resveratrol, and vitamin C) were the matter of previous investigations on their role in dental implant osseointegration. Available data suggest that severe vitamin D deficiency or even the presence of established osteoporosis led to a higher implant failure rate [29,31] or to a worse BIC [34,35]. In osteoporotic rats, vitamin D depletion led to a significant decrease in BIC in the cortical area. Moreover, rats that received vitamin D showed a similar BIC to the control group [34]. Animal studies on vitamin D and osseointegration confirmed that the early stages of bone healing could be significantly influenced by vitamin D status [35–40]. In humans, Mangano et al. [29,31] reported a clear trend toward an increased incidence of early implant failures within the group with lower serum 25(OH)D levels. In particular, the authors reported 11.1% EDIF in patients with serum 25(OH)D < 10 ng/mL (severe vitamin D deficiency), 4.4% for those with 25(OH)D between 10 and 30 ng/mL, and 2.9% in patients with normal vitamin D status.

Moreover, Wagner et al. [30] showed that osteoporosis has a significant negative influence on marginal bone loss around implants and that vitamin D supplementation counteracts the marginal bone loss, with overall results of beneficial effects on the peri-implant bone formation.

Vitamin D deficiency commonly occurs in the general population. This hormone has a crucial function in skeletal mineralization, but also plays an important role in immunity and inflammatory response, increasing anti-inflammatory cytokines and decreasing pro-inflammatory ones [55].

Bashutski et al. [56] showed that, in vitamin D-deficient individuals, minimal benefits could be obtained from periodontal surgery along with an impaired post-surgical healing. Vitamin D could have other effects on osseointegration that are more related to soft tissue healing and marginal seals around implants, together with an effect on resistance against bacterial infections of the peri-implant sulcus. Also, topical applications of vitamin D were used for implant coating, showing some beneficial effects in animals, such as a reduction in crestal bone loss and an increase of BIC [57]. However, several critical issues persist regarding the use of vitamin D in enhancing osseointegration, particularly concerning its mechanism(s) of action, the influence of different serum 25(OH)D levels, and the recommended dosages required to significantly improve dental implant success rate.

Also, vitamin C deficiency may have a role in tissue healing and stability around dental implants. This micronutrient plays an important role in the biosynthesis of collagen, which is an important component of connective tissue of the gingiva, peri-implant mucosa, and alveolar bone [58]. These effects were confirmed by Li et al. [47], who found that vitamin C supplementation improved postoperative wound healing following dental implant surgery. Moreover, protective effects of this intervention on bone health could be expected, as vitamin C could hinder the effects of oxidative stress in promoting bone resorption and consequently reducing bone strength [59], although this hypothesis is not yet confirmed. However, the role of vitamin C supplementation in the general population, as well as in patients receiving dental implants, might be significantly affected by lifestyle, including smoking habits and diet, two factors that affect wound healing times. Furthermore, plasma ascorbic acid concentrations are not reported in clinical practice [60].

With regard to resveratrol, Casarin et al. [43] investigated its role on bone healing of calvarial defects in rats through messenger RNA (mRNA) quantification of bone morphogenetic protein (BMP)-2, BMP-7, osteopontin (OPN), bone sialoprotein (BSP), osteoprotegerin (OPG), and receptor activator of nuclear factor kappa B (NF-κB) ligand (RANKL). Gene expression analysis showed a higher expression of *BMP-2* ($p = 0.011$), *BMP-7* ($p = 0.049$), and *OPN* ($p = 0.002$) genes in the resveratrol-fed group than in the control group.

Ribeiro et al. [42] reported encouraging data about biomechanical retention and peri-implant bone formation in resveratrol-fed rats exposed to cigarette smoking inhalation, supporting a positive role of this substance in controlling different osteogenic mechanisms. Their gene expression analysis demonstrated that lower RANKL/OPG levels were detected in rats receiving resveratrol, as well as in non-smoking animals, when compared to animals exposed to smoking and receiving placebo. Both studies on resveratrol confirmed the substantial improvement in implant stability, by modulating the expression of genes involved in bone regulatory processes. However, the main limitation of findings supporting resveratrol, as well as magnesium, is the availability of animal studies only.

However, considering the results of our research, several micronutrients are non-authorized or even not considered by the "EU Register on nutrition and health claims" on the basis of current scientific evidence.

Major nutrients involved in skeletal health include calcium, phosphorus, vitamin D, magnesium, and potassium, but other micronutrients and trace elements such as boron, selenium, iron, zinc, and copper also impact bone metabolism. Information on the influence of such "minor" elements coming from studies on nutrient depletion and studies on osseointegration is still lacking.

5. Conclusions

Our scoping review overall demonstrated a lack of data about the effects of micronutrients and nutraceuticals on osseointegration of dental implants, although, for some of them, such as vitamin D, there was a clear association among their deficit, reduced osseointegration, and increased early implant failure incidence in both animal and human studies.

Some micronutrient deficiencies are supposed to increase oxidative stress and inflammation and to affect collagen structure and bone mineralization. For these reasons, it would be desirable that further studies investigate the hypothesis of an influence of micronutrients and nutraceuticals on dental implant osseointegration and long-term success, as well as the opportunity of a diet integration to enhance peri-implant wound healing, bone healing, and peri-implant tissue stability. However, data for many micronutrients that might modulate bone metabolism are lacking, and dosing regimens for dietary supplements that improve dental implant osseointegration are not defined according to available findings; furthermore, safety issues remain to be carefully investigated. In conclusion, our findings support an ancillary role of vitamin D, in patients with vitamin D deficiency, as well as vitamin C supplementation, in facilitating the success of the dental implant surgery.

Supplementary Materials: The following are available online at http://www.mdpi.com/2072-6643/12/1/268/s1, Table S1: Search strategy.

Author Contributions: Conceptualization, L.N., A.M., S.M., L.G., and G.I.; methodology, L.N., A.M., S.M., M.P., M.A., S.L., G.T., M.B., and G.I.; writing—original draft preparation, L.N., A.M., M.P., M.A., G.C., and G.I.; writing—review and editing, L.N., A.M., M.P., M.A., S.L., G.T., M.B., G.C., L.G., and G.I.; funding acquisition, L.G. and G.I. All authors read and agreed to the published version of the manuscript.

Funding: The authors would like to acknowledge the Vanvitelli per la Ricerca (VALERE) program for the allocation of funding that aims to publish University of Campania "Luigi Vanvitelli" research products.

Conflicts of Interest: The authors declare no conflict of interest. The funders had no role in the design of the study; in the collection, analyses, or interpretation of data; in the writing of the manuscript, or in the decision to publish the results.

References

1. Zarb, G.A.; Albrektsson, T. Osseointegration—A requiem for the periodontal ligament? *Int. J. Periodontol. Restor. Dent.* **1991**, *11*, 88–91.
2. Goiato, M.C.; Dos Santos, D.M.; Santiago, J.F., Jr.; Moreno, A.; Pellizzer, E.P. Longevity of dental implants in type IV bone: A systematic review. *Int. J. Oral Maxillofac. Surg.* **2014**, *43*, 1108–1116. [CrossRef]
3. Esposito, M.; Hirsch, J.M.; Lekholm, U.; Thomsen, P. Biological factors contributing to failures of osseointegrated oral implants. (I). Success criteria and epidemiology. *Eur. J. Oral Sci.* **1998**, *106*, 527–551. [CrossRef]
4. Esposito, M.; Thomsen, P.; Ericson, L.E.; Lekholm, U. Histopathologic observations on early oral implant failures. *Int. J. Oral Maxillofac. Implants* **1999**, *14*, 798–810.
5. Huynh-Ba, G.; Friedberg, J.R.; Vogiatzi, D.; Ioannidou, E. Implant failure predictors in the posterior maxilla: A retrospective study of 273 consecutive implants. *J. Periodontol.* **2008**, *79*, 2256–2261. [CrossRef] [PubMed]
6. Sverzut, A.T.; Stabile, G.A.; de Moraes, M.; Mazzonetto, R.; Moreira, R.W. The influence of tobacco on early dental implant failure. *J. Oral Maxillofac. Surg.* **2008**, *66*, 1004–1009. [CrossRef] [PubMed]
7. Urban, T.; Kostopoulos, L.; Wenzel, A. Immediate implant placement in molar regions: Risk factors for early failure. *Clin. Oral Implants Res.* **2012**, *23*, 220–227. [CrossRef] [PubMed]
8. WHO Micronutrients. Available online: https://www.who.int/nutrition/topics/micronutrients/en/ (accessed on 27 December 2019).
9. Iolascon, G.; Gimigliano, R.; Bianco, M.; De Sire, A.; Moretti, A.; Giusti, A.; Malavolta, N.; Migliaccio, S.; Migliore, A.; Napoli, N.; et al. Are Dietary Supplements and Nutraceuticals Effective for Musculoskeletal Health and Cognitive Function? A Scoping Review. *J. Nutr. Health Aging* **2017**, *21*, 527–538. [CrossRef]
10. Montalvany-Antonucci, C.C.; Zicker, M.C.; Oliveira, M.C.; Macari, S.; Madeira, M.F.M.; Andrade IJr Ferreira, A.V.; Silva, T.A. Diet versus jaw bones: Lessons from experimental models and potential clinical implications. *Nutrition* **2018**, *45*, 59–67. [CrossRef]

11. Aguirre, J.I.; Akhter, M.P.; Kimmel, D.B.; Pingel, J.; Xia, X.; Williams, A.; Jorgensen, M.; Edmonds, K.; Lee, J.Y.; Reinhard, M.K.; et al. Enhanced alveolar bone loss in a model of non-invasive periodontitis in rice rats. *Oral Dis.* **2012**, *18*, 459–468. [CrossRef]
12. Kametaka, S.; Miyazaki, T.; Inoue, Y.; Hayashi, S.I.; Takamori, A.; Miyake, Y.; Suginaka, H. The effect of ofloxacin on experimental periodontitis in hamsters infected with Actinomyces viscosus. *J. Periodontol.* **1989**, *60*, 285–291. [CrossRef] [PubMed]
13. Fujita, Y.; Maki, K. High-fat diet induced periodontitis in mice through lipopolysaccharides (LPS) receptor signaling: Protective action of estrogens. *BMC Obes.* **2016**, *3*, 1–9. [CrossRef] [PubMed]
14. De Albuquerque Taddei, S.R.; Madeira, M.F.M.; de Abreu Lima, I.L.; Queiroz-Junior, C.M.; Moura, A.P.; Oliveira, D.D.; Andrade, I., Jr.; da Glória Souza, D.; Teixeira, M.M.; da Silva, T.A. Effect of Lithothamnium sp and calcium supplements in strain- and infection-induced bone resorption. *Angle Orthod.* **2014**, *84*, 980–988. [CrossRef] [PubMed]
15. Barò, M.A.; Rocamundi, M.R.; Viotto, O.J.; Ferreyra, R.S. Alveolar wound healing in rats fed on high sucrose diet. *Acta Odontol. Latinoam.* **2013**, *26*, 97–103.
16. Tricco, A.C.; Lillie, E.; Zarin, W.; O'Brien, K.K.; Colquhoun, H.; Levac, D.; Moher, D.; Peters, M.D.; Horsley, T.; Weeks, L.; et al. PRISMA Extension for Scoping Reviews (PRISMA-ScR): Checklist and Explanation. *Ann. Intern. Med.* **2018**, *169*, 467–473. [CrossRef]
17. Dermience, M.; Lognay, G.; Mathieu, F.; Goyens, P. Effects of thirty elements on bone metabolism. *J. Trace Elem. Med. Biol.* **2015**, *32*, 86–106. [CrossRef]
18. Farley, J.R.; Wergedal, J.E.; Baylink, D.J. Fluoride directly stimulates proliferation and alkaline phosphatase activity of bone-forming cells. *Science* **1983**, *222*, 330–332. [CrossRef]
19. Dommisch, H.; Kuzmanova, D.; Jönsson, D.; Grant, M.; Chapple, I. Effect of micronutrient malnutrition on periodontal disease and periodontal therapy. *Periodontology 2000* **2018**, *78*, 129–153. [CrossRef]
20. Bushinsky, D.A.; Riordon, D.R.; Chan, J.S.; Krieger, N.S. Decreased potassium stimulates bone resorption. *Am. J. Physiol. Ren. Physiol.* **1997**, *272*, F774–F780. [CrossRef]
21. Ornstrup, M.J.; Harsløf, T.; Sørensen, L.; Stenkjær, L.; Langdahl, B.L.; Pedersen, S.B. Resveratrol Increases Osteoblast Differentiation in Vitro Independently of Inflammation. *Calcif. Tissue Int.* **2016**, *99*, 155–163. [CrossRef]
22. Choi, H.K.; Kim, G.J.; Yoo, H.S.; Song, D.H.; Chung, K.H.; Lee, K.J.; Koo, Y.T.; An, J.H. Vitamin C Activates Osteoblastogenesis and Inhibits Osteoclastogenesis via Wnt/β-Catenin/ATF4 Signaling Pathways. *Nutrients* **2019**, *11*, 506. [CrossRef]
23. Kim, H.-N.; Lee, J.-H.; Jin, W.J.; Lee, Z.H. α-Tocopheryl Succinate Inhibits Osteoclast Formation by Suppressing Receptor Activator of Nuclear Factor-kappaB Ligand (RANKL) Expression and Bone Resorption. *J. Bone Metab.* **2012**, *19*, 111–120. [CrossRef]
24. Myneni, V.D.; Mezey, E. Regulation of bone remodeling by vitamin K2. *Oral Dis.* **2017**, *23*, 1021–1028. [CrossRef]
25. Yamaguchi, M. Nutritional factors and bone homeostasis: Synergistic effect with zinc and genistein in osteogenesis. *Mol. Cell. Biochem.* **2012**, *366*, 201–221. [CrossRef] [PubMed]
26. Yamaguchi, M. Role of nutritional zinc in the prevention of osteoporosis. *Mol. Cell. Biochem.* **2010**, *338*, 241–254. [CrossRef] [PubMed]
27. Cruz, A.C.C.; Cardozo, F.T.G.S.; Magini, R.S.; Simões, C.M.O. Retinoic acid increases the effect of bone morphogenetic protein type 2 on osteogenic differentiation of human adipose-derived stem cells. *J. Appl. Oral Sci.* **2019**, *27*, e20180317. [CrossRef]
28. Fratoni, V.; Brandi, M.L. B vitamins, homocysteine and bone health. *Nutrients* **2015**, *7*, 2176–2192. [CrossRef]
29. Mangano, F.; Ghertasi Oskouei, S.; Paz, A.; Mangano, N.; Mangano, C. Low serum vitamin D and early dental implant failure: Is there a connection? A retrospective clinical study on 1740 implants placed in 885 patients. *J. Dent. Res. Dent. Clin. Dent. Prospects* **2018**, *12*, 174–182. [CrossRef] [PubMed]
30. Wagner, F.; Schuder, K.; Hof, M.; Heuberer, S.; Seemann, R.; Dvorak, G. Does osteoporosis influence the marginal peri-implant bone level in female patients? A cross-sectional study in a matched collective. *Clin. Implant Dent. Relat. Res.* **2017**, *19*, 616–623. [CrossRef] [PubMed]
31. Mangano, F.; Mortellaro, C.; Mangano, N.; Mangano, C. Is Low Serum Vitamin D Associated with Early Dental Implant Failure? A Retrospective Evaluation on 1625 Implants Placed in 822 Patients. *Mediat. Inflamm.* **2016**, *2016*, 5319718. [CrossRef] [PubMed]

32. Fretwurst, T.; Grunert, S.; Woelber, J.P.; Nelson, K.; Semper-Hogg, W. Vitamin D deficiency in early implant failure: Two case reports. *Int. J. Implant Dent.* **2016**, *2*, 24. [CrossRef] [PubMed]
33. Bryce, G.; MacBeth, N. Vitamin D deficiency as a suspected causative factor in the failure of an immediately placed dental implant: A case report. *J. R. Naval Med. Serv.* **2014**, *100*, 328–332.
34. Liu, W.; Zhang, S.; Zhao, D.; Zou, H.; Sun, N.; Liang, X.; Dard, M.; Lanske, B.; Yuan, Q. Vitamin D supplementation enhances the fixation of titanium implants in chronic kidney disease mice. *PLoS ONE* **2014**, *9*, e95689. [CrossRef]
35. Zhou, C.; Li, Y.; Wang, X.; Shui, X.; Hu, J. 1,25Dihydroxy vitamin D3 improves titanium implant osseointegration in osteoporotic rats. *Oral Surg. Oral Med. Oral Pathol. Oral Radiol.* **2012**, *114*, S174–S178. [CrossRef] [PubMed]
36. Wu, Y.Y.; Yu, T.; Yang, X.Y.; Li, F.; Ma, L.; Yang, Y.; Liu, X.G.; Wang, Y.Y.; Gong, P. Vitamin D3 and insulin combined treatment promotes titanium implant osseointegration in diabetes mellitus rats. *Bone* **2013**, *52*, 1–8. [CrossRef]
37. Akhavan, A.; Noroozi, Z.; Shafiei, A.A.; Haghighat, A.; Jahanshahi, G.R.; Mousavi, S.B. The effect of vitamin D supplementation on bone formation around titanium implants in diabetic rats. *Dent. Res. J.* **2012**, *9*, 582–587. [CrossRef]
38. Dvorak, G.; Fügl, A.; Watzek, G.; Tangl, S.; Pokorny, P.; Gruber, R. Impact of dietary vitamin D on osseointegration in the ovariectomized rat. *Clin. Oral Implants Res.* **2012**, *23*, 1308–1313. [CrossRef]
39. Kelly, J.; Lin, A.; Wang, C.J.; Park, S.; Nishimura, I. Vitamin D and bone physiology: Demonstration of vitamin D deficiency in an implant osseointegration rat model. *J. Prosthodont. Implant Esthet. Reconstr. Dent.* **2009**, *18*, 473–478. [CrossRef]
40. Belluci, M.M.; Giro, G.; Del Barrio, R.A.L.; Pereira, R.M.R.; Marcantonio, E., Jr.; Orrico, S.R.P. Effects of magnesium intake deficiency on bone metabolism and bone tissue around osseointegrated implants. *Clin. Oral Implants Res.* **2011**, *22*, 716–721. [CrossRef]
41. Del Barrio, R.A.; Giro, G.; Belluci, M.M.; Pereira, R.M.; Orrico, S.R. Effect of severe dietary magnesium deficiency on systemic bone density and removal torque of osseointegrated implants. *Int. J. Oral Maxillofac. Implants* **2010**, *25*, 1125–1130.
42. Ribeiro, F.V.; Pimentel, S.P.; Corrêa, M.G.; Bortoli, J.P.; Messora, M.R.; Casati, M.Z. Resveratrol reverses the negative effect of smoking on peri-implant repair in the tibia of rats. *Clin. Oral Implants Res.* **2019**, *30*, 1–10. [CrossRef] [PubMed]
43. Casarin, R.C.; Casati, M.Z.; Pimentel, S.P.; Cirano, F.R.; Algayer, M.; Pires, P.R.; Ghiraldini, B.; Duarte, P.M.; Ribeiro, F.V. Resveratrol improves bone repair by modulation of bone morphogenetic proteins and osteopontin gene expression in rats. *Int. J. Oral Maxillofac. Surg.* **2014**, *43*, 900–906. [CrossRef] [PubMed]
44. Pimentel, S.P.; Casarin, R.C.; Ribeiro, F.V.; Cirano, F.R.; Rovaris, K.; Haiter Neto, F.; Casati, M.Z. Impact of micronutrients supplementation on bone repair around implants: microCT and counter-torque analysis in rats. *J. Appl. Oral Sci.* **2016**, *24*, 45–51. [CrossRef] [PubMed]
45. Takahashi, T.; Watanabe, T.; Nakada, H.; Sato, H.; Tanimoto, Y.; Sakae, T.; Kimoto, S.; Mijares, D.; Zhang, Y.; Kawai, Y. Improved Bone Micro Architecture Healing Time after Implant Surgery in an Ovariectomized Rat. *J. Hard Tissue Biol.* **2016**, *25*, 257–262. [CrossRef] [PubMed]
46. Watanabe, T.; Nakada, H.; Takahashi, T.; Fujita, K.; Tanimoto, Y.; Sakae, T.; Kimoto, S.; Kawai, Y. Potential for acceleration of bone formation after implant surgery by using a dietary supplement: An animal study. *J. Oral Rehabil.* **2015**, *42*, 447–453. [CrossRef] [PubMed]
47. Li, X.; Tang, L.; Lin, Y.F.; Xie, G.F. Role of vitamin C in wound healing after dental implant surgery in patients treated with bone grafts and patients with chronic periodontitis. *Clin. Implant Dent. Relat. Res.* **2018**, *20*, 793–798. [CrossRef]
48. Chrcanovic, B.R.; Albrektsson, T.; Wennerberg, A. Smoking and dental implants, a systematic review and meta-analysis. *J. Dent.* **2015**, *43*, 487–498. [CrossRef]
49. Arora, M.; Schwarz, E.; Sivaneswaran, S.; Banks, E. Cigarette smoking and tooth loss in a cohort of older Australians, the 45 and Up Study. *J. Am. Dent. Assoc.* **2010**, *141*, 1242–1249. [CrossRef]
50. Dietary Supplement Products & Ingredients. FDA. Available online: https://www.fda.gov/food/dietary-supplements/dietary-supplement-products-ingredients (accessed on 27 December 2019).

51. DeFelice, S. The NutraCeutical Revolution: Fueling a Powerful, New International Market. Presented at the Harvard University Advanced Program in Biomedical Research Management and Development, Como, Italy; 1989. Available online: https://fimdefelice.org/library/the-nutraceutical-revolution-fueling-a-powerful-new-international-market/ (accessed on 27 December 2019).
52. Zeisel, S.H. Regulation of "nutraceuticals". *Science* **1999**, *285*, 1853–1855. [CrossRef]
53. Aronson, J.K. Defining 'nutraceuticals': Neither nutritious nor pharmaceutical. *Br. J. Clin. Pharmacol.* **2017**, *83*, 8–19. [CrossRef]
54. Fulgoni, V.L., III; Keast, D.R.; Auestad, N.; Quann, E.E. Nutrients from dairy foods are difficult to replace in diets of Americans: Food pattern modeling and an analyses of the National Health and Nutrition Examination Survey 2003–2006. *Nutr. Res.* **2011**, *31*, 759–765. [CrossRef] [PubMed]
55. Nastri, L.; Guida, L.; Annunziata, M.; Ruggiero, N.; Rizzo, A. Vitamin D modulatory effect on cytokines expression by human gingival fibroblasts and periodontal ligament cells. *Minerva Stomatol.* **2018**, *67*, 102–110. [CrossRef] [PubMed]
56. Bashutski, J.D.; Eber, R.M.; Kinney, J.S.; Benavides, E.; Maitra, S.; Braun, T.M.; Giannobile, W.V.; McCauley, L.K. The impact of vitamin D status on periodontal surgery outcomes. *J. Dent. Res.* **2011**, *90*, 1007–1012. [CrossRef] [PubMed]
57. Salomó-Coll, O.; Maté-Sánchez de Val, J.E.; Ramírez-Fernandez, M.P.; Hernández-Alfaro, F.; Gargallo-Albiol, J.; Calvo-Guirado, J.L. Topical applications of vitamin D on implant surface for bone-to-implant contact enhance: A pilot study in dogs part II. *Clin. Oral Implants Res.* **2016**, *27*, 896–903. [CrossRef]
58. Boyera, N.; Galey, I.; Bernard, B.A. Effect of vitamin C and its derivatives on collagen synthesis and cross-linking by normal human fibroblasts. *Int. J. Cosmet. Sci.* **1998**, *20*, 151–158. [CrossRef] [PubMed]
59. DePhillipo, N.N.; Aman, Z.S.; Kennedy, M.I.; Begley, J.P.; Moatshe, G.; LaPrade, R.F. Efficacy of Vitamin C Supplementation on Collagen Synthesis and Oxidative Stress After Musculoskeletal Injuries: A Systematic Review. *Orthop. J. Sports Med.* **2018**, *6*, 2325967118804544. [CrossRef]
60. DiPietro, S.G.L.A. Factors affecting wound healing. *J. Dent. Res.* **2010**, *89*, 219–229.

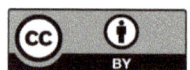

© 2020 by the authors. Licensee MDPI, Basel, Switzerland. This article is an open access article distributed under the terms and conditions of the Creative Commons Attribution (CC BY) license (http://creativecommons.org/licenses/by/4.0/).

MDPI
St. Alban-Anlage 66
4052 Basel
Switzerland
Tel. +41 61 683 77 34
Fax +41 61 302 89 18
www.mdpi.com

Nutrients Editorial Office
E-mail: nutrients@mdpi.com
www.mdpi.com/journal/nutrients

www.ingramcontent.com/pod-product-compliance
Lightning Source LLC
LaVergne TN
LVHW070544100526
838202LV00012B/378